THE PSYCHOLOGY OF TEAM SPORTS

Ronnie Lidor

Keith Page Henschen

Editors

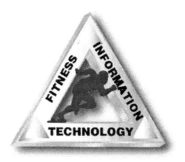

Fitness Information Technology, Inc. • P.O. Box 4425 • Morgantown, WV 26504-4425 • USA

© Copyright 2003, by Fitness Information Technology, Inc.

Library of Congress Card Catalog Number: 2002116144

ISBN: 188529332X

Copyeditor: Sandra Woods
Cover Design: Jamie Pein
Cover Photo: © SportsChrome
Managing Editor: Geoff Fuller
Production Editor: Jackie Pauley
Proofreader: Jessica McDonald
Indexer: Jessica McDonald
Printed by: Publishers' Graphics
10 9 8 7 6 5 4 3 2 1

Fitness Information Technology, Inc.
P.O. Box 4425, University Avenue
Morgantown, WV 26504 USA
800.477.4348
304.599.3483 phone
304.599.3482 fax
Email: fit@fitinfotech.com
Web Site: www.fitinfotech.com

CONTENTS

Part I: Introduction

Part II: Looking for Empirical Support: Related Issues for Team Sports

Part III: Performing Sport Psychology within the Team: Specific Sports

Contents

TABLES AND FIGURES

ACKNOWLEDGMENTS

We have been working on the *Psychology of Team Sports* for about two years. The book represents the theoretical as well as the applied fruits of professionals from North America, Europe, and Asia who are involved in team sport activities. Our main goal was to create a relevant body of knowledge for sport psychologists, coaches, and athletes. We believe that the information presented by the contributors to this book will help sport psychologists and coaches better prepare their teams for practices, competitions, and games.

We would like to thank all the individuals who contributed chapters to this book; their cooperation and enthusiasm were key factors in its completion. In addition, we would like to thank Professor Robin Vealey and Professor Edward F. Etzel for providing us with fruitful comments and advice during the preparation of the book. Their suggestions undoubtedly helped to improve the quality of the book.

We would like to acknowledge the work done by Dinah Olswang, from the Ribstein Center for Sport Medicine Sciences and Research at the Wingate Institute for Physical Education and Sport (Israel). Her assistance in preparing each chapter was instrumental in our goal of achieving uniformity throughout the book, and her efforts are deeply appreciated. In addition, we would like to thank the research committee at the Zinman College of Physical Education and Sport Sciences for providing financial support throughout the preparation of the book.

Finally, we would like to thank Andrew Ostrow, our publisher, and Geoff Fuller, the managing editor of the book, from Fitness Information Technology, for their valuable advice, encouragement, and support during each phase of the preparation of this project.

PREFACE

The "second coming" of Michael Jordan to the National Basketball Association, the second one during his remarkable career, has attracted the attention of people all over the world. Basketball addicts, sport fans, and individuals who usually do not spend time watching sport programs on TV all were waiting impatiently for Michael Jordan's words: "I am back." This player has elevated the game of basketball to the highest level of human performance. He is considered by many to be the greatest ball player to ever play the game. His extraordinary physical and mental abilities enabled him to achieve the highest level of proficiency in his sport.

However, Michael Jordan was not alone. He achieved his greatness as an individual athlete while part of a team of players who worked as hard as they could to achieve the best they were capable of. Without the professional and mental assistance, cooperation, and support of these individuals he could not have reached the peak of his game. This is why the psychological and social relationships that Jordan developed with his teammates were of as much interest as his professional relationship with them. The public at large, as well as athletes, coaches, team managers, and the media, were eager to know what was going on inside the teams which Jordan played for. They understood the complexity existing within the structure of a team sport; they realized the difficulties each player on the team had to cope with while being required to cooperate with others on and off the court. This complexity is even greater when the team has to deal with a "mega star" of such a caliber as Michael Jordan. If we add the roles of the coaching staff, the medical and the management personnel, and the media individuals involved in a sport team, we increase this complexity even more. Athletes in team sports must not only develop solid relationships among the other members of the team, but also with these "external" individuals who provide them with the appropriate stage for fulfilling their potential and achieving their best. To put it simply, it is hard to be part of a team sport.

It is also hard, however, to work with team sports. The complexity that emerges within a team sport makes it more difficult for those working with a team sport on a regular basis to apply an approach, concept, or strategy, on and off the court or field. There are many aspects to consider while working with a team of individuals in sport settings. Among these are technical (e.g., individual and team fundamentals), tactical (e.g., how to play offensively and how to build a strong defense), physical (e.g., how to improve the fitness level of each player), and psychological (e.g., how to be mentally prepared for practices and games) aspects. Each one can affect the effort of the team and the outcome of this effort. Combinations of these aspects can also affect the performance and the final results obtained by the team. It could be a combination of the physical and the tactical aspects of the team that affects its performance. It could be instead that a mixture of technical and the mental aspects of the team influence its poor (or good) performance. It is very difficult, and sometimes impossible, to cope effectively with the multi-faceted combinations that might affect the performance of a team in sport settings. Psychology of Team Sports focuses solely on psychological aspects of team sports. It is true that many texts in sport and exercise psychology have discussed the psychological aspects of team sports. However, these sources also provide information on psychological aspects of individual sport activities as well as recreational and health-oriented programs. This book discusses only psychological issues related to team sport activities, on and off the court or field. The book presents a three-phase model (Chapter 1) that attempts to assist sport psychologists and coaches in reducing the complexities they face while working with team sports. This model can be applied in a variety of team activities, such as baseball, basketball, ice hockey, soccer, and others. The following chapters in the book, Chapters 2 to 12, provide sport psychologists and coaches with theoretical (Chapters 2 to 7) and practical (Chapters 8 to 12) advice. The book presents not only major theoretical concepts related to team sport activities but also experiences shared by sport psychologists who have worked for long periods of time with professional clubs and teams as well as national teams.

We know that it is difficult to cover all the psychological aspects related to team sports. We attempted in this book to elaborate upon those issues that are most relevant to sport psychologists working with team sports. We selected issues that are important for a variety of team activities, for females and males, and for beginner and experienced athletes.

Some of the ideas presented in the book can be used not only by sport psychologists but also by coaches and athletes. Our assumption was that the psychological aspects of a team practicing and competing on a regular basis are as important as the physical, technical, and tactical aspects. We believe that the psychological aspect is positively related to the other aspects of the team in its drive for success. It is our hope that sport psychologists as well as other individuals working with team sports will apply some of the ideas introduced in the book. These ideas can be utilized in various ways according to the team's goals, structure, and spirit.

The Editors,
Ronnie Lidor, Ph.D.
Keith Henschen, Ph.D.

PART I

INTRODUCTION

CHAPTER 1

Working With Team Sports: Applying a Holistic Approach

Ronnie Lidor and Keith Henschen

John Wooden, former head coach of the record-setting UCLA basketball team that won 10 national championships in 12 years, used to tell his players that failing to prepare is preparing to fail (Wooden, 1988). The Pyramid of Success, an influential motivational and instructional device that he developed, reflects the idea that in order to achieve success in any kind of team sport activity, one has to do the best that one is capable of—but within the structure, spirit, and goals of the team (Wooden, 1980).

Team sports are one of the most popular professional and recreational activities around the globe. When a person walks near a park, court, gym, or other sport or recreational facility, he or she will probably see some kind of ball game being played or some other team or group activity. About two decades ago the famous zoologist, Desmond Morris, described the game of soccer as a unique worldwide religious ceremony. He argued that

> it is no longer [soccer] accompanied by high-pitched laughter, but by deep groans, shouts and roars from manly throats. It is now a serious endeavor, with every move dissected and debated in earnest tones, the whole ritual elevated to the level of a dramatic social event. (D. Morris, 1981, p. 8)

This observation can be applied to other team sport activities as well, such as baseball, basketball, volleyball, team-handball, and even track and field (which can be classified as an individual team sport; see chapter 12).

People of all ages enjoy team activities. They regularly invest a great number of hours in improving their skills—some do so because they want to compete at the highest level of proficiency, as John Wooden's players did, and others, just for the fun of it. Recreational as well as professional players are required to work not only on their physical skills, but also on their emotional and mental skills.

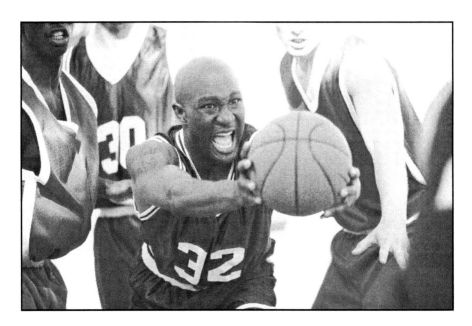

*Sport today has become increasingly aggressive and serious –
even during casual pickup games.*

Regardless of the motives for participation in team sports, an individual is required to be physically and mentally prepared. There is certainly no lack of technical guidelines in the sport and physical education literature on how to enhance basic technical and physical fundamentals in all kinds of team sport activities (e.g., Philipp & Wilkerson, 1990). Players and coaches are aware of the necessity of facilitating their motor behaviors, such as responses, reactions, and anticipation during a game or match. However, do they know how to develop emotional, mental, and social skills related to team activities? Can they discover intervention programs, strategies, and techniques that have been successfully used by sport psychologists and sport counselors in their practical experiences with individual athletes involved in team sport activities?

Sport psychologists, coaches, and players can probably find some relevant and useful information on these issues in the general texts on sport and exercise psychology that have been published during the last two decades (e.g., Bull, 1993; Gill, 2000; Hardy, Jones, & Gould, 1996; T. Morris & Summers, 1995; Murphy, 1995; Singer, Hausenblas, & Jannelle, 2001; Tenenbaum, 2001; Weinberg & Gould, 1999). However, most of these books provide an equal focus on individual and team sport activities. The strategies and techniques elaborated upon in these psychological sources can be used in both types of activities, but only after being modified by the coach and the player. In addition to these general sport psychology texts, in which related topics on team sport performances are also included, there are specific psychology sources for specific sports, such as baseball (Dorfman & Kuehl, 1989) and basketball (Mikes, 1987). These sources provide sport psychologists, coaches, and athletes with useful practical knowledge on how to work in team sports. However, these sources do not provide the scientific background relevant to certain issues related to team sports, such as team cohesion, emotions in sport, and attentional control.

Therefore, an attempt was made in this book to combine psychological, developmental, and instructional perspectives relating solely to team sport activities, from both scientific and applied perspectives, in order to provide a unique body of knowledge for coaches, players, sport psychologists, and professional consultants. The main purpose of this book is to provide those professionals who are involved in team sport activities, on and off the court or field, with theoretical—and, more importantly, applied—guidance on how to enhance cognitive, emotional, mental, and social behaviors of players who are active in team sport activities. In addition, we have tried to provide good advice from experienced applied psychologists who have been working for many years with elite athletes and teams at the top level of human competition.

Our preliminary assumption is that it is not an easy task to work in team sports, not for the sport consultant and also not for other professionals assisting the team, such as biomechanist, exercise physiologist, or weight-lifting instructor. A team sport is composed of two or more individuals playing together with a clear goal to excel. To achieve this goal, the members of the team should work together within a structured hierarchy, and they should be willing to accept this hierarchy. In a typical sport situation, the members of a team are required to practice together regularly in order to improve not only their group skills but also their individual ones. In addition, each member of the team is an independent individual who comprises a variety of characteristics, some of which are genetically inherent, some of which have been acquired through life experience. There are characteristics that are unique to only one individual, and others that are shared among members of the team.

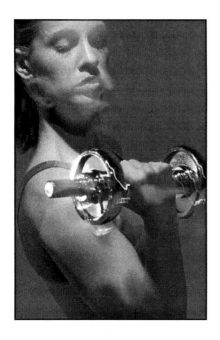

Every team member must consider and respect the team as a whole during every team-related activity – even independent workouts.

To improve the psychological support given to team sports, we should take into account the difficulties that were previously mentioned as well as the complexities that emerge from the actual work with a team of individuals in sport. There are so many factors involved in the psychology of team sports that one may think it is almost impossible to provide a group of individuals in a team with the appropriate preparation. Among these factors, we can outline those that are internal and related to the framework and structure of the team (e.g., leading athletes within the team, veteran versus upcoming players) as well as those that are related to the relationship between the team and external factors, such as the team opponents (i.e., on-court factors) and the media (i.e., off-court factors). (A variety of factors that are potentially involved in the study of team sport activities are reported in detail in chapter 2.)

Working With Team Sports: A 3-Phase Approach

In order to assist sport psychologists in their attempts to overcome the difficulties that exist in working with team sports and to reduce the complexity the sport psychologist faces while working with individuals within a team, we would like to propose a 3-phase approach that can be used while working with team sports.

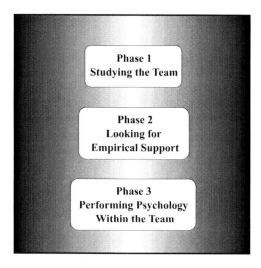

Figure 1. Working with team sports: A 3-phase approach

This approach can be applied in team sports, such as baseball, basketball, ice hockey, and soccer, and in individual team sports, such as track and field. The 3-phase approach, as seen in Figure 1, includes the following phases:

During Phase 1, Studying the Team, sport psychologists are asked to study carefully, systematically, and patiently the team with which they are going to work. Before conducting any intervention program or taking any other practical step, sport psychologists must collect information about the team. For example, they must understand how the coach runs the team and determine the relationships among the coaching staff. They should also identify the key players and the "superstars" of the team. However, because the sport psychologists are not with the team all the time, they have to gather the information from a variety of sources. When the consultants stay with the team, they can observe the players' and the coaches' behaviors, talk with them, and administer psychological and sociological questionnaires. When the teams are away and the sport psychologists do not accompany them, they have to use other sources of information gathering, such as videos of the team's performance and audio cassettes on which players are recorded sharing their perspectives on their own or the teams performances. In some cases, sport psychologists can look at archival data to obtain information related to the team's past performances. This "historical" information may assist sport psychologists to better understand how the team reacted in the past under similar conditions. If all the pieces of information emerging from different sources (as presented in Figure 2) are incorporated effectively, then useful information can be incorporated by the consultants to aid them in facilitating the psychological services they administer to the team.

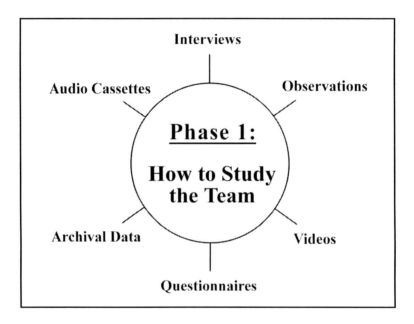

Figure 2. Studying the team: How to collect information

After the consultants gather the relevant information, carefully study the team, and are about to develop a plan of action, they should then move to Phase 2: Looking for Empirical Support. We frankly advise professionals working with team sports to consult the scientific literature in sport and exercise psychology and search for the best solutions for their needs. Because of the difficulties and complexities that professionals face while working with team sports, they have to rely on scientific sources to enhance their decision-making processes. It is recommended that professionals apply findings that have emerged from scientific inquiries when working with team sports. Laboratory and field investigations in sport and exercise psychology on topics such as intervention strategies and techniques for performance enhancement, team cohesion, team leadership, attentional control, and emotional regulations can provide useful guidance for sport psychologists on how to work with team sports.

However, we all know that on many occasions we are not able to apply scientific findings to the field. In fact, it is sometimes very difficult to take a good idea that is presented in a journal article, a chapter in a book, or a book and apply it in practical settings "as is." This is the reason why "how to" sport psychology texts have been published recently (Andersen, 2000; Tenenbaum, 2001). The main purpose of these texts is to demonstrate how sport psychologists work with athletes. It is demonstrated in Andersen's (2000) and Tenenbaum's (2001) collections of experiences of applied sport psychologists that there is more than one way to effectively administer psychological services to athletes. Among the topics presented in these texts the sport psychologist can find some material related to team sport activities as well.

The transition between the theoretical searching process that is undertaken in Phase 2 of our 3-phase approach and the selection of appropriate regulations, strategies, and techniques used by sport psychologists occurs in Phase 3. During Phase 3, Performing Psychology Within the Team, the sport consultants are required to match the selected techniques with the team's conditions, spirit, and structure, among other factors. They have to understand that the scientific literature has not yet provided some issues with clear evidence of what sport consultants should do while working with team sports. For example, issues such as working with "superstars," handling off-court behavior of young talented athletes, the coach-athlete-sport psychologist relationship, sport psychologists working with female versus male athletes, and the athletes-media relationship can have a crucial impact on the final success of a team. It can be difficult to find clear-cut guidelines in the sport psychology literature, both the scientific and the applied, on how to deal with some of these issues. Moreover, it is almost impossible to study these issues under well-controlled experimental manipulations. Thus, sport psychologists have to use their common sense and life experience, combined with knowledge acquired from reading sport-related psychology literature, in order to establish an appropriate plan of psychological support. Therefore, in Phase 3 they should develop readiness and solve problems within the team by implementing a combined approach: using ideas introduced to them in the literature and adapting those ideas according to their own needs.

We have attempted to organize the chapters in this book within the framework of our 3-phase approach. In Part II we placed six chapters that provide sport psychologists with ideas that can help them apply phases 1 and 2 of our approach. We believe that the foundation of any consultation process should be based on both good methodology and empirical background. The stronger the methodological and scientific foundations (e.g., Phase 1 of our approach), the better the conceptual understanding of what should be done by the sport psychologist with and within the team. In other words, sport psychologists who work in team sports should have a solid idea of how to study team sport activities (see, for example, chapter 2) and a good theoretical background of issues related to team sport activities (see, for example, chapters 4, 5, 6, and 7).

Nevertheless, we also believe that sport psychologists have to use their common sense and own experiences to conduct an effective psychological readiness program. That is why we asked five well-known and experienced sport psychologists from North America and Europe to share with us their knowledge and perspectives on how to conduct sport psychology within a team. Thus, the chapters included in Part III (i.e., chapters 8 to 12) are meant to assist sport psychologists in better planning Phase 3 of our approach. All these chapters reflect the experiences of psychologists working at the highest levels of sport competition.

The Structure of the Book

This book consists of three parts. Part I, *Introduction*, contains one chapter. Chapter 1 (Ronnie Lidor and Keith Henschen), "Working With Team Sports: Applying a Holistic Approach," is divided into two parts and provides a conceptualized introduction for the book. In the first part, a 3-phase approach to working with team sports is introduced. The approach includes three phases, as follows: (a) studying the team, (b) looking for empirical support, and (c) performing psychology within the team. The authors provide their view on how such an approach can assist consultants to cope efficiently with the difficulties and complexities they face while working with a team of different personalities, egos, abilities, etc., in sport settings. In addition, the authors explain how the chapters of the book are organized according to the 3-phase approach. In the second part of chapter 1, background for each chapter included in the book (i.e., chapters 2 to 12) is provided.

Part II, *Looking for Empirical Support: Related Issues for Team Sports*, contains six chapters. This part introduces a variety of psychological issues related to team sport activities. These issues — methodological, ethical, instructional, cognitive, and social — reflect a multi-faceted structure of sport team activity. To understand the psychology of team activities, a variety of components should be considered; the greater number of components considered, the better the conceptual understanding. Each of the topics discussed in chapters 2 to 7 can be applied to almost every team sport activity. Every coach, player, and sport psychologist working in team sports should take these topics into consideration.

Chapter 2 (Gershan, Tenenbaum, and Barry Kirker), "Methodological Principles in the Study of Behaviors in Team Sports: An Example of Aggressive Acts in Ice Hockey and Basketball," develops a methodology for the investigation of behaviors in team sports. Usually dynamic and open skilled, team sports involve a variety of actions that are aimed at exhibiting superiority over the opponent. In addition, team sports vary in many aspects, such as rules, amount of physical contact, number of players, and culture. To study the antecedents and consequences of team athletes' behaviors, a sound research methodology is needed. This methodology consists of all the factors (personal, external, and environmental) that may to some degree determine athletes' behaviors. The authors outline the possible sources of team sport athletes' behaviors, along with the observational techniques that are aimed at their measurement. The authors then suggest how these observations should be triangulated and later interpreted with respect to the foundation theory and the concepts underlying this methodology. After the model is suggested, the methodology is presented by using examples of investigating aggressive behaviors in ice hockey and basketball.

Chapter 3 (Richard D. Gordin), "Ethical Issues in Team Sports," contains a brief overview of common ethical issues to be considered when a coach, a sport psychologist, and any other sport professional works with team sports. The chapter contains three parts. In the first part, the author presents the ethical guidelines established by the Association for the Advancement of Applied Sport Psychology (AAASP) and the American Psychological Association (APA). These guidelines are of particular interest to both the coach and the sport psychologist. In the second part, several anecdotes from the author's 25 years of experience as an applied sport psychologist are reported. In the third part, practical recommendations for sport psychologists who work with team sports are provided.

Chapter 4 (Ronnie Lidor and Robert N. Singer), "Preperformance Routines in Self-Paced Tasks: Developmental and Educational Considerations," examines developmental and educational considerations related to attaining proficiency in preperformance routines in young athletes who are involved in ballgame activities. These considerations reflect the psychological foundations needed to master self-paced skills as performed in real-game situations. The authors argue that in order to benefit from a particular routine, an individual ideally should experience and master it during the initial process of acquiring skill in any self-paced event. The chapter provides a brief overview of the literature on the use of preperformance routines in sport and discusses the psychological factors contributing to success in self-paced skills executed in team sports. Based on the analysis of the psychological characteristics of self-paced tasks, the authors suggest that a learning strategy be used as part of the technical guidelines introduced to the learners at the initial phase of the learning process. By doing so, an instructional link between the technique of the learned skill and the psychological characteristics of the skill is created. This link may provide coaches in team sports with the knowledge of how to assist athletes in acquiring strategies and techniques that might contribute to a desirable preparatory routine.

Chapter 5 (Paul A. Estabrooks and Paul W. Dennis), "The Principles of Team Building and Their Applications to Team Sports," focuses on practical team-building intervention strategies. The authors examine the conditions necessary to consider "a collective of individuals" as "a group." They define group cohesion in terms of its dynamic and multidimensional nature, taking into account the empirical evidence associated with cohesion and sport. Step-by-step instructions regarding the implementation of both direct and indirect team-building intervention are provided for both the coach and the sport psychologist.

Chapter 6 (Cal Botterill and Tom Patrick), "Understanding and Managing Emotions in Team Sports," presents a general discussion of emotions in sport, derived primarily from the literature within sport psychology. Of importance to athletes, coaches, and sport psychologists is achieving an improved understanding of how emotions affect performance and how they can be managed more effectively. The authors present suggestions for improving emotional preparation and emotional management based on their collective practical experiences, through their work with elite athletes and coaches in Canada. The authors attempt to provide coaches and sport psychologists with some practical tools to optimizing performance in team sports.

Chapter 7 (Gloria Balague), "Gender Differences When Working With Men's and Women's Teams," presents the view that the role of a sport psychologist when consulting, traveling, and generally working with individual athletes is often complex. Each individual athlete is unique and therefore requires special treatment. Even more complex, though, is the role of the sport psychologist working with team sports. The reason for this observation is that subtle interpersonal issues combine with individual factors and may influence the performance of the whole group. Men's and women's athletic teams may be faced with similar problems, but how the teams deal with these problems is usually different. The author discusses some of the interpersonal issues and individual factors that frequently occur in athletic teams, according to gender. In addition, she suggests some interventions that are effective in remedying these issues and problems — again according to gender.

Part III, *Performing Sport Psychology Within the Team: Specific Sports*, contains five chapters. Each chapter focuses on a different team sport: Basketball, soccer, baseball, and ice hockey are the topics of chapters 8, 9, 10, and 11, respectively. Track and field is the topic of the last chapter in this part, chapter 12. The first four sports are "ballgame" activities that share similar characteristics, such as defensive and offensive structures within the team, special roles for each player within the team, a specific procedure of scoring, etc. The only sport that is not specifically a team sport is track and field. Track and field is considered an individual team sport, containing 23 athletic events in which individual athletes are trying to achieve the best by competing against each other. In a typical track event, such as the 100 m sprint or the 5000 m run, and a field event, such as the long jump or the shot put, athletes stand by themselves without the ability to use teammates to provide them with support in their attempts to achieve first place. They rely only on their own physical and psychological abilities. However, being part of a track-and-field team means that one is part of a team. In other words, track and field can be also considered as a team sport, and it shares some of the characteristics of a team sport, such as basketball, soccer, and baseball. This is the reason that track and field is included in this part.

Chapter 8 (Keith Henschen and David Cook), "Working With Professional Basketball Players," reflects the notion that professional basketball players, such as NBA players, are not special individuals, but rather individuals with special physical talents who are forced to live a little differently than the rest of us. Moreover, it is the rare professional player who effectively deals with the pressure put on him or her both on and off the court. This chapter points out that team interventions are normally not accepted, the cooperation of coaches is crucial to the success of the sport psychologist, and individual counseling with players and coaches should be the primary method of service delivery. Among the issues frequently encountered by the sport psychologist working at the professional level outlined in the chapter are slumps, motivation, use of free of time, fragile egos, and cliques. Other topics discussed by the authors are dealing with the media, handling success and failure, and handling trades. The authors provide some words of advice based on their personal experiences.

Chapter 9 (Aidan Moran), "Improving Concentration Skills in Team Sport Performance: Focusing Techniques for the Soccer Players," discusses the ability to focus mental effort on what is most important in any situation, while ignoring distractions. This cognitive ability is widely regarded as a vital determinant in any success at all levels of sport competition. The purpose of this chapter is to elaborate upon some of the issues related to focusing skills, such as the mechanisms underlying this skill, the reasons that athletes seem to lose their focus so easily, and the ways in which athletes should be trained to improve their attentional skills. The chapter combines research findings on attentional skills with practical implications for the sport psychologist. More specifically, six practical focusing techniques are illustrated in the case of soccer players.

Chapter 10 (Tom Hanson and Ken Ravizza), "Issues for the Sport Psychology Professional in Baseball," is based on the notion that baseball players typically report that 80% or more of their performance is determined by mental and emotional factors. The authors believe that the task of sport psychology professionals is to educate players and coaches on the fundamentals of the mental game and provide a structure of support for them as they develop their abilities to use their thoughts and emotions to their best advantage. Following a presentation of their three main objectives, the authors emphasize the importance of understanding the nature of baseball and the process of building relationships, credibility, and trust within the team. The authors conclude the chapter with common issues they have addressed when working with baseball players.

Chapter 11 (Peter Haberl and Len Zaichkowsky), "The U.S. Women's Olympic Gold Medal Ice Hockey Team: Optimal Use of Sport Psychology for Developing Confidence," provides a psychological report on one sport team, namely the U.S. Women's 1998 Olympic gold medal ice hockey team. The authors choose one sport psychology concept, namely, confidence, to share with professionals and students who have an interest in sport psychology, in order to give an idea of what a sport psychologist does in the world of ice hockey. Instead of discussing the myriad of skills and techniques they used in their work with the team, they focus on this one aspect of psychological interventions. First, the authors present the history of the ice hockey team, and then they elaborate on the importance of confidence in sport. After describing some of the theoretical concepts of confidence in sport, the authors explain in detail how they used modeling in various forms to build confidence among the members of the team. The authors suggest the use of verbal persuasion as a source of confidence that can be used effectively by the coach as well as by teammates.

Chapter 12 (Ralph A. Vernacchia), "Working With Individual Team Sport: The Psychology of Track and Field," addresses the salient aspects of "working with an individual team sport," such as track and field. To give prospective sport psychology consultants a better understanding of the social and performance climate of track and field, the author provides an overview of the culture, politics, and mentality of track and field. The author emphasizes the concept of team dynamics, with particular focus on the importance of social support and the recognition of gender differences as key components of the team-building process. He postulates a track-and-field specific model for the design and implementation of an educational mental skills program in track and field.

The book represents the fruits of not only the applied, but also the theoretical, work of individuals from all over the world who are involved in team sport activities. Their theoretical inquiries as well as practical experiences create a relevant body of knowledge for sport psychologists, coaches, and athletes. We believe that the chapters included in this book will provide sport psychologists and coaches with some of the assistance they need to ready their teams for practices, competitions, or games. This readiness program should help the coaches and, in turn, the athletes, to overcome some of the major emotional, mental, and even physical obstacles they have to face while competing with their opponents at high levels of human performance.

Tenenbaum and Kirker (2002, chapter 2 in this book) argue that "team sports are usually dynamic, open-skill types, and involve many activities that are aimed at exhibiting superiority over the opponents. Team sports vary in many aspects, such as values, number of players, and culture" (p. 21). To develop readiness for practice and competition in such an environment, competent sport psychologists should move smoothly from Phase 2 to Phase 3 of the approach suggested in this chapter (see Figure 3). They have to rely on empirical support, however, and also to use their common sense at the same time.

To put it simply, sport psychologists have to use a holistic approach while working with team sports. This holistic approach should reflect a strong scientific foundation as well as good common sense.

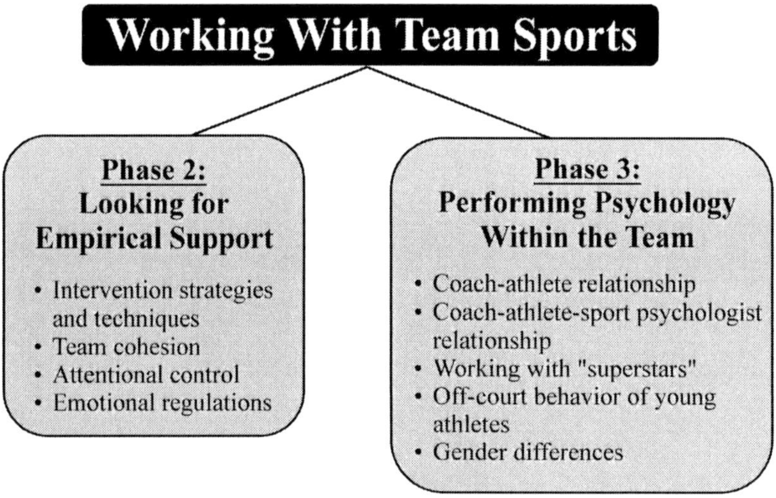

Working With Team Sports

Phase 2:
Looking for
Empirical Support

- Intervention strategies and techniques
- Team cohesion
- Attentional control
- Emotional regulations

Phase 3:
Performing Psychology
Within the Team

- Coach-athlete relationship
- Coach-athlete-sport psychologist relationship
- Working with "superstars"
- Off-court behavior of young athletes
- Gender differences

Figure 3. Working with team sports:
The transition between phases 2 and 3

For example, although team sports are classified as activities performed in an open environment (i.e., a variable and unpredictable environment [Schmidt & Lee, 1999; Schmidt & Wrisberg, 2000]), athletes are required to perform well also under closed settings (i.e., a stable and predictable environment [Schmidt & Lee, 1990; Schmidt & Wrisberg, 2000]), such as free-throw shots in basketball and an 11-m kick in soccer, as presented in Figure 4. This means that the athletes should be exposed not only to mental preparation programs used before the game, but also to specific mental preperformance routines that are executed just a few seconds before the execution of a self-paced task (see chapter 4 for more information related to the usage of preperformance routines in self-paced tasks in team sports). A well-developed readiness program should reflect the needs of an individual athlete within a team activity.

We attempt in this book to present not only "straightforward" research findings that have emerged from laboratory and field investigations, but also some views of sport consultants who have been working with team sports over a long period. It is our hope that the psychological issues elaborated upon throughout the book will enable the enhancement of coaching, teaching, consultation, and application in team sports.

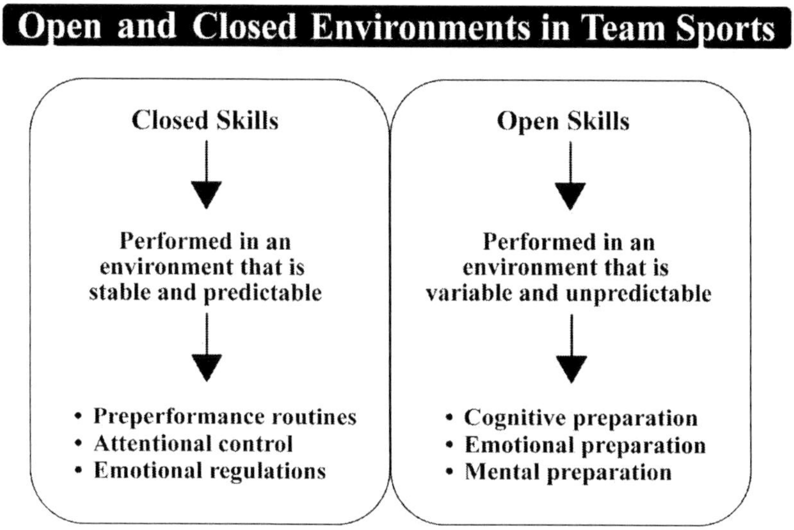

Open and Closed Environments in Team Sports

Closed Skills	Open Skills
↓	↓
Performed in an environment that is stable and predictable	Performed in an environment that is variable and unpredictable
↓	↓
• Preperformance routines • Attentional control • Emotional regulations	• Cognitive preparation • Emotional preparation • Mental preparation

Figure 4. Open and closed environments in team sports

References

Andersen, M. B. (Ed.). (2000). *Doing sport psychology.* Champaign, IL: Human Kinetics.

Bull, S. J. (1993). *Sport psychology: A self-help guide.* Edinburgh: The Crowood Press.

Dorfman, H. A., & Kuehl, K. (1989). *The mental game of baseball: A guide to peak performance.* South Bend, IN: Diamond Communications.

Gill, D. L. (2000). *Psychological dynamics of sport and exercise* (2nd ed.). Champaign, IL: Human Kinetics.

Hardy, L., Jones, G., & Gould, D. (1996). *Understanding psychological preparation for sport: Theory and practice of elite performers.* Chichester: Wiley.

Mikes, J. (1987). *Basketball fundamentals: A complete mental training guide.* Champaign, IL: Leisure Press.

Morris, D. (1981). *The soccer tribe.* London: Jonathan Cape.

Morris, T., & Summers, J. (Eds.) (1995). *Sport psychology: Theory, applications and issues.* Brisbane: Wiley.

Murphy, S. M. (Ed.). (1995). *Sport psychology interventions.* Champaign, IL: Human Kinetics.

Philipp, J. A., & Wilkerson, J. D. (1990). *Teaching team sports: A coeducational approach.* Champaign, IL: Human Kinetics.

Schmidt, R. A., & Lee, T. D. (1999). *Motor control and learning: A behavioral emphasis* (3rd ed.). Champaign, IL: Human Kinetics.

Schmidt, R. A. & Wrisberg, C. A. (2000). *Motor learning and performance: A problem-based learning approach* (2nd ed.). Champaign, IL: Human Kinetics.

Singer, R. N., Hausenblas, H. A., & Janelle, C. M. (Eds.) (2001). Handbook of sport psychology (2nd ed.). New York: Wiley.

Tenenbaum, G. (Ed.). (2001). *The practice of sport psychology.* Morgantown, WV: Fitness Information Technology.

Tenenbaum, G., & Kirker, B. (2002). *Methodological principles in the study of behaviors in team sports: An example of aggressive acts in ice hockey and basketball.* In R. Lidor & K. Henschen (Eds.), Psychology of team sports (pp. 21-55). Morgantown, WV: Fitness Information Technology.

Weinberg, R. S., & Gould, D. (1999). *Foundations of sport and exercise psychology* (2nd ed.). Champaign, IL: Human Kinetics.

Wooden, J. R. (1980). *Practical modern basketball* (2nd ed.). New York: Wiley.

Wooden, J. R. (1988). *They call me coach.* Chicago: Contemporary Books.

PART II

LOOKING FOR EMPIRICAL SUPPORT: RELATED ISSUES FOR TEAM SPORTS

CHAPTER 2

Methodological Principles in the Study of Behaviors in Team Sports: An Example of Aggressive Acts in Ice Hockey and Basketball

Gershon Tenenbaum and Barry Kirker

Abstract

In this chapter we have developed a methodology for the investigation of behaviors in team sports. Team sports are usually dynamic, open skill-types, and they involve many actions that are aimed at exhibiting superiority over the opponents. Team sports vary in many aspects, such as rules, number of players, and culture. In order to study the antecedents and consequences of team athletes' behaviors, a sound research methodology is required. This methodology consists of all the factors (personal, external, and environmental) that may determine to some degree athletes' behaviors. We outline the possible sources of team sport athletes' behaviors, along with the observational techniques that are aimed at their measurement, and postulate how these observations should be triangulated and later interpreted with respect to the foundation theory and concepts underlying this methodology. After postulating the model, the methodology is presented by using an example of investigating aggressive behaviors in ice hockey and basketball.

Science and Methodological Framework for Studying Behaviors in Team Sports

Observation is guided by and presupposes theory. Theories can be established as true or probably true in the light of observational evidence. Theories are construed as speculative and tentative conjectures or guesses freely created by the human intellect in an attempt to overcome problems encountered by previous theories and to give an adequate account of the behavior of some aspects of the world or universe. Once proposed, speculative theories are to be rigorously and ruthlessly tested by observation and experiment. Theories that fail to stand up to observational and experimental tests must be eliminated and replaced by further speculative conjectures. Science progresses by trial and error, by conjectures and refutations. Only the fittest theories survive. Although it can never be legitimately said of a theory that it is true, it can hopefully be said that it is the best available, that it is better than anything that has come before (Chalmers, 1982, p. 38).

Chalmers's views on science imply that a theory must guide the methodology, which determines the nature and procedures of any investigation. We use this view to investigate the antecedents, intentions, and consequences of behaviors that occur in competitions of team sports. The theory enables the establishment of hypotheses and accordingly sets up a methodology aimed at investigating them.

The operational definitions (i.e., instrumentation and observational techniques) are then selected so that data can be collected for analysis. Behaviors that occur during competition may result from a variety of sources. These can be intrapersonal, interpersonal, intergroup, intragroup, and environmental, as well as other sources like family and peers. One may consider these sources as affecting behaviors separately and integratively. Once factors associated with behaviors are identified, typologies and taxonomies of behaviors can be developed so that systematic observations can be conducted. Observations can be in the form of coding behaviors, measurement through introspective questionnaires, structured or nonstructured interviews, or all of them integratively. Archival data; expert opinions; and reflections of players, referees, spectators, coaches, and others are recommended to triangulate the sources of evidence. When the data are in a form suitable for analysis, a unique methodology should be applied in which the reflections, judgments, and introspective data are integrated to edit specific events that were filmed and/or recorded. A traditional research methodology is of little value in this respect. A holistic and systematic methodology that is aimed at all possible factors of behaviors' influence and that considers both quantitative and qualitative data and interpretations is preferable. The outlines of such a methodology are introduced in Figure 1.

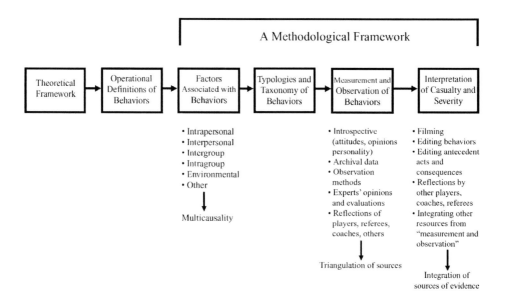

Figure 1. A theory-based methodology for studying behaviors in team sports

Every research plan starts with a theoretical conceptualization of the questions and variables that constitute it. The theoretical concept outlines the relations among the variables and the causality and effects of one, or a few, upon the others. Once the variables are identified, an operational definition is assigned to each of them so that these variables can be measured. Each measure, whether of an introspective or objective nature, should share acceptable reliability and validity properties. Factors associated with behaviors of athletes in team sports can be intrapersonal, interpersonal, intergroup, intragroup, environmental, and others. Usually one should consider all of these factors integratively, so that typologies and taxonomies can be developed. Once taxonomies of possible behaviors and their sources are established, the measurement and observations can be determined. As Figure 1 shows, the observations can be of different natures and use different sources, so that triangulation of perspectives can be integrated into a holistic perspective.

To illustrate this methodological perspective in team sport, an investigation of aggressive and assertive behaviors in team sports is introduced. The theories, which postulate the variables of such behaviors, are described briefly, and then the stages of methodology development in line with Figure 1 are introduced in more detail. It is not the aim here to demonstrate classical research methodology, results, and discussion. Instead, we introduce the principles of the holistic approach we advocate to use in similar investigations.

Psychological Theories on Aggression in Sport

At least three theories offer explanations for the antecedents and occurrence of aggressive behaviors in sport: instinct theory, frustration-aggression (F-A) theory, and social learning theory.

Freud originally proposed that humans are born with aggressive instincts, which stem from innate biological drives. These brutish instincts are suppressed by social values and norms, but must be fulfilled. Aggression stems from a venting of built-up energy or emotions. Sport provides a positive and socially acceptable outlet for these natural tendencies. Once these energies are released, humans need no longer be aggressive until another buildup takes place and release is again required (see Cox, 1990). The main problem with this theory is that observations have shown that aggression leads to further aggression (Pfister, 1982).

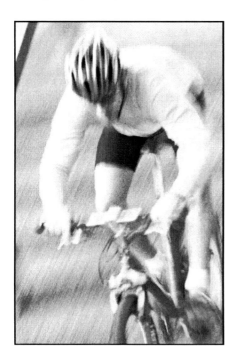

Being part of a team means regular workouts, which provide regular release for pent-up energy.

The frustration-aggression theory (Dollard, Miller, Doob, Mourer, & Sears, 1939) claims that aggression is always a consequence of frustration. The theory was later revised (Berkowitz, 1978) and suggested that frustration (i.e., anything that blocks the attainment of a goal) does not always produce aggressive behaviors, but rather heightens one's predisposition toward aggression. Frustration causes anger that leads to aggression when aggressive cues exist. In sport, such cues can appear in the form of verbal utterances by spectators, minor rule infringements from opponents, or errors from officials. Typically, the strongest instigation of aggression is directed toward the source of frustration (Cox, 1990). Observations have indicated that in many instances, frustrated individuals tend to reduce their efforts or withdraw from an activity rather than become aggressive (Anshel, 1994; Cox, 1990).

Social learning theory (Bandura, 1979) postulates that aggression is a learned response. In sport, aggression is acquired and maintained through the process of modeling, vicarious learning, and directly experienced learning. This theory also claims that, whether realized indirectly or directly, aggressive behaviors seem to be mostly rewarding. Research has consistently demonstrated the modeling effect in youth sport (Cox, 1990; Goldstein, 1983; Smith, 1982; Thirer, 1993).

A number of psychologists have suggested that sport, due to its competitive and emotion-raising nature, fosters aggression (Cox, 1990; Lefebrve & Passer, 1974; Leith, 1982; Russell & Drewry, 1976). However, few theorists have related to differences across sporting situations in regard to aggression. Aggression seems to have no place in certain individual sport (e.g., shooting and archery), whereas it is particularly associated with fast, open-skilled team sport. Further, it may be that different processes contribute to aggressive behavior in team competition but not in individual competition.

With each team sport having its own culture, aggression may manifest itself in different ways and amounts in different team sports. There is a lack of empirical basis for generalizing aggressive behaviors across team sports. Ice hockey has been the most widely researched sport in relation to sports violence and aggressive play, and it is usually cited as the standard for aggression in sport. This is linked to the widespread belief that aggression in ice hockey is a normalized and necessary feature of the game (Anshel, 1994; Goldstein, 1983; LeUnes & Nation, 1989; Smith, 1980, 1982; Vaz, 1977).

To reliably investigate the causes of aggressive behaviors in team sport, a methodological framework was developed in accordance with the principles outlined in Figure 1. Next we present how the methodological framework was established.

A Methodological Framework for the Study of Aggressive Behaviors in Team Sports

The first stage in establishing a methodological framework for investigation consists of providing the operational definitions of the behaviors in the study. When such a definition lacks consistent agreement, the researcher ought to establish such a definition. Aggression according to Husman and Silva (1984) and Cox (1990) is a term that lacks consistent and clear definition. However, the most salient features of aggressive acts are the "intent" and "severity" of the aggressive acts. Accordingly, aggression, the infliction of an aversive stimulus (either physical or nonphysical) during forceful and intense action, upon one person by another or by him- or herself, is a behavior committed with intent to injure (Anshel, 1994; Bakker, Whiting, & Van der Brug, 1995; Cox, 1990, LeUnes & Nation, 1989; Widmeyer & Birch, 1984). It is the concept of intent that is the defining characteristic of aggressive behavior and that distinguishes aggressive acts from other outwardly similar behaviors that are forceful assertive acts (Connelly, 1988; Cox, 1990). However, severity is an associated variable that also contributes to the term's clarification. In sport, forceful acts range from minor (e.g., a player trying to win possession) to more severe (e.g., players striking each other or an official).

Aggression involves nonphysical behaviors as well as physical contact. Verbal utterances and gestural acts, for example, can be behaviors intended to harm. However, typically, nonphysical behaviors are less severe than physical actions. The term violence is often used interchangeably with that of aggression (Goldstein, 1983). Although violent behavior is also aggressive behavior, violence involves the most severe aggressive acts, such as players' brawling or attacks on officials. Finally, although a person can direct aggressive behavior upon himself or herself, typically aggressive acts are inflicted on other people.

Assertiveness, like aggressiveness, involves forceful behavior and intensity of action, physical or otherwise. However, the intent behind assertive behavior is not to hurt another, but rather only to be active and determined and to establish dominance (Anshel, 1994; Connelly, 1988; Cox, 1990; Husman & Silva, 1984; LeUnes & Nation, 1989; McGuire, Courneya,

Widmeyer, & Carron, 1992). Assertive behavior, typically integral to sporting endeavor, can result in injury, but such physical or psychological harm is incidental to the play. Due to the absence of malicious intent, assertive behavior is typically less severe than aggressive behavior.

The second methodological concern relates to the factors that are associated with behaviors such as aggressive acts. The extensive research in this field offers factors that are intrapersonal, interpersonal, intragroup, intergroup, and environmental and that bear some relationship with sport aggression. The relevance of a wide theoretical perspective (i.e., a holistic view) to the underlying processes of aggression is evident with the varying nature of potential casual variables behind these behaviors (i.e., aggressive acts). Alone, each variable may not be sufficient for causation. The probability of an aggressive act's occurrence is higher when certain factors interact. Brief examples for the various factors related to aggressive acts are presented below.

Intrapersonal Factors

Frustration, the central variable in the F-A theory, can be considered an emotional experience that is related to aggressive behaviors. Whether frustration is a variable that itself initiates aggression, or whether the important variables are arousal and other meaningful cues for aggression that occur simultaneously, is uncertain. Research has shown what common sense suggests, that aggression is more likely to occur when a player is aroused (Bar-Eli & Tenenbaum, 1989; Cox, 1990). In line with the F-A theory, arousal may be a readying mechanism for aggression. The highly aroused (angered) person is in a state in which the presence of an aggressive stimulus could trigger an aggressive response. Arousal may interact with many of the factors addressed in this section, and thus, many of the factors that follow could be considered aggressive cues or triggers.

The values placed on the various expected reinforcements and punishments also play a part in this context (Bandura, 1979; Silva, 1980). Considerable anecdotal evidence suggests that both situational expectancies and generalized expectancies influence whether a player will commit aggressive behavior in sport (Silva, 1980). Players' perception of an opponent's behavior may also be an important determinant of aggression. If players perceive that the intent of an opponent is to inflict harm or otherwise commit an offense in relation to them, then players are more likely to be aggressive in response. Conversely, if players perceive that an opponent does not intend to hurt them, they may hold back on displaying aggressive behavior (Cox, 1990). Specifically, perceptions of blame may play a role in players' attribution of aggressive behavior.

Players also vary in their attitudes towards aggression in sport. Furthermore, players may hold a different attitude in regard to aggression in sport in general than they do in regard to aggression in their own sport, where they are very familiar with specific scenarios and situations (Bakker et al., 1995; Silva, 1980). Individual differences may also play a part in regard to seemingly trivial or nonsense factors that have been reported to operate as special triggers or cues for aggression. For some individuals, aggressive cues may be as subtle as the color of a team's uniform. Frank and Gilovich (1988) found that more penalties were conceded by professional American sports teams that wore black uniforms than by those who did not. Further, when teams changed to black uniforms, they experienced an increase in penalties incurred.

Interpersonal Factors

Linked to players' perceptions of opponents' behavior and natural hostile reactions, research in both sport and nonsport settings suggests that it is a typical response for persons to retaliate against those who have aggressed against them (Harrell, 1980; LeUnes & Nation, 1989; Russell, 1974). The F-A theory suggests that the strongest instigation for aggression will be toward the source of the frustration. An opponent's behavior is probably the most common source of a player's aggressive action. Harrell further suggested that retaliatory aggression is hostile in nature, often dysfunctional, and primarily frustration induced.

The decisions of officials are likely to be important factors in sports aggression. In most games, officials make errors or ignore rule violations (Bar-Eli & Tenenbaum, 1989; Mark, Bryant, & Lehman, 1983), and in doing so they upset and frustrate players. The more serious the consequences and the more flagrant the error, the more likely an officiating error is to lead to aggressive behavior (Mark et al., 1983). Also, the aggression of fans due to poor officiating decisions is a mediating variable that influences players' reactions.

The relationship between officiating style and aggression is particularly important. Bakker et al.'s research (1995) consisted of several studies and concluded that most punishable events had to do with the referee and the way he or she was controlling the game. It has been suggested that officials who keep tight control over a game can prevent instrumental aggression (Mark et al., 1983). It is equally plausible that a less authoritarian officiating style would lead to reduced aggression, as players would be less likely to display hostile aggression toward an official who was pleasant and not interfering.

In addition to the attention given to aggression by the media and fans, coaches, teammates, and even family can encourage the aggressive behaviors of a player (Anshel, 1994; Luxbacher, 1986; Smith, 1980, 1982). Coaches do encourage players to use aggression as a strategy for intimidation and success (Luxbacher, 1986; Smith, 1982). Smith (1982) suggested that coaches encourage aggressive play "both for what it symbolizes (gameness and strong character) and for its utility in winning games and enhancing players careers" (p. 305). He also cited some evidence for the fact that coaches tend to choose players on the basis of size and toughness (among other attributes).

Intergroup Factors

The amount and/or nature of previous intergroup (and within that, interpersonal) encounters may be an important mediator of aggression between opposing teams and players. Widmeyer and McGuire (1997) found a relationship between frequency of competition and aggression in professional ice hockey. There was a significant difference in the number of aggressive penalties per game when teams competed more frequently (seven or eight times a season) than when teams competed less frequently (3 times a season). These findings were attributed to the existence of historical grudges between players as a result of previous conflicts that were of increased likelihood when regular competitive interaction occurred.

Widmeyer and McGuire (1997) also found a reduction in the amount of aggression when games were of more critical importance (i.e., play-off games), suggesting an interaction effect between frequency of competition and efforts to minimize penalization and "adventurous play" in critical games. Other research has also found critical game situations to have a mediating effect on the occurrence of aggressive play (Cox, 1990). Conceding a penalty or losing a player in critical clashes or critical situations within a game can prove decisive in determining the eventual match or league winner. Specifically, it has been found that aggression is more prevalent among losing teams than winning ones (Cox, 1990; LeFebvre & Passer, 1974; Martin, 1976; Russell & Drewry, 1976) and is related to a team's league standing or game importance. Furthermore aggression increases as game score differential increases (LeFebvre & Passer, 1974; Russell & Drewry, 1976; Widmeyer & McGuire, 1997).

A relatively large amount of research has considered time gone or period in the game as a factor (Bakker et al., 1995; Widmeyer & Birch, 1984). Widmeyer and Birch (1984) suggested that for learned reasons, players strategically commit higher amounts of aggression in the earlier stages of sporting contests. Widmeyer and Birch (1984) noted that the amount of aggression committed early in a contest, enabling a player or team to "get on top" or to "take the early initiative," may be offset by aggression occurring later in a game by frustrated and/or revenge-seeking teams that are losing. Consistent with other studies, and in contrast to Widmeyer and Birch (1984), Bar-Eli and Tenenbaum (1989) found that major rule violations (aggressive behavior) in basketball were more likely to occur in the second half of games than in the first half.

It is unclear whether players are more aggressive playing at home or playing away. It was believed that visiting teams display more aggressive behaviors than home teams do (LeFebvre & Passer, 1974). However, Russell and Drewry (1976) found no difference between the amount of aggressive play between home and visiting ice hockey teams, and Kelly and McCarthy (1979) found that home teams were in fact more aggressive than visiting teams. As part of a recent study offering a multivariate explanation of home advantage in professional ice hockey, McGuire et al. (1992) considered aggression in association with Courneya and Carron's (1992) framework for game location research. This model considers the main features of playing at home to be crowd support, lack of travel, familiarity, and benefit of doubt from officials. McGuire et al., 1992 concluded that a home advantage did exist and that the advantage was mediated by aggressive behavior.

Intragroup Factors

It has been theorized that the notion of "deindividuation" may play a role in the occurrence of aggression in team sport (LeUnes & Nation, 1986). This is a process whereby the existence of group dynamics leads to a decrease in personal identity and responsibility for behavior and an increase in conformity to group norms. Shields, Bredemeiser, Gardner, and Bostrom (1995) found that collective or team norms in terms of a "moral atmosphere" influence players' propensity for aggressive behavior. Shields et al., 1995 considered aggression particularly in relation to team cohesion and leadership style (coach), both of which were found to mediate the relationship between team norms and player attitudes towards aggression as well as player expectations about peer aggression.

Environmental Factors

Spectators may play a significant role in the aggressive behavior of players. Although it is debatable as to whether the "mere presence" of spectators at sporting events affects players (Cox, 1990; Russell, 1981b; Russell & Drewry, 1976), it seems clear that certain spectators' behaviors can affect a player's mood and behavior during a game. Spectator behavior of an antisocial, abusive nature can lead to overly elevated player arousal levels (Thirer, 1993). Additionally, the cheering and encouragement of overly forceful and often aggressive play can foster and reinforce the occurrence of aggressive acts. Spectators' behaviors can lead to on-field aggression in both direct (i.e., directly affecting a player's mood or behavior) and indirect ways (i.e., affecting an official's or opponent's mood or behavior).

Fans' influence does not always work to their team's advantage. Interestingly, Thirer and Rampey (1979) found that home basketball teams were more negatively affected by the antisocial behavior of spectators than were the visiting teams. They also found that the closer and more crowded the spectators were, the more influence they could have (Thirer & Rampey, 1979). Previously, Russell and Drewry (1976) found that crowd size was positively related to aggression in the Canadian Ice Hockey League. Physical factors, such as hot and noisy conditions, and individual differences in player anxiety and concentration can be mediating variables on crowd effects (LeUnes & Nation, 1986; Thirer & Rampey, 1979).

The relationship between player behavior and spectator behavior is not unidirectional. Complex bidirectional relationships exist; fans influence the behavior of players, but also players' actions influence the fans' behavior. Moreover, at times the interaction between fans and players can be as dynamic as that between players (Goldstein, 1983). For example, the mood and subsequent aggressive behavior of spectators at ice hockey games has been found to be affected by aggressive play on the ice (Russell, 1981b). In turn, the increased spectator hostility was found likely to contribute to higher aggression levels among players and so on (i.e., a regressing circular relationship). Nevertheless, literature that treats fan and athlete aggression as if it has identical causes (e.g., Goldstein, 1983) is problematic. There are clearly a number of differing factors involved in fan hooliganism and not just rough play among players.

In nonsport settings, heat has been found to have a curvilinear relationship with aggressive acts (LeUnes & Nation, 1986). However, a linear relationship has been found in sport. Reifman, Larrick, and Fein (1991) found a positive relationship between temperature and the number of baseball batters hit by a pitch per game.

Finally, off-field factors that may increase a player's propensity for aggressive action in the sports arena must be noted. Research in other areas of psychology has identified a number of variables from an individual's life experiences, particularly from childhood, that increase the likelihood that a person will commit aggressive acts in a variety of settings (Bandura, 1979; Cox, 1990; Le Unes & Nation, 1986). It can be assumed that events and attitudes occurring outside of sport competition may have some effect on an athlete's on-field mood and behavior, even considering the ability of today's professional athlete to mentally limit the influence of such events.

Other Factors

There are a number of other factors considered to have some relationship to aggressive behavior in sport. They include perceptions of an opponent's capabilities (Anshel, 1994); sexual abstinence (Gelso & Mandracchia, 1983); birth order of a player (Russell, 1981a); withholding of an aggressive response or a buildup of emotion (Schneider & Eitzen, 1986); a player's level of moral reasoning (Bredemeier, 1985); age or experience of a player (Shields et al., 1995); the position of a player, defensive or offensive (Bakker et al., 1995); geographical distance between teams (Bakker et al., 1995); amount of time spent on the bench (Shields et al., 1995); and degree of body contact between players in the game (Bakker et al., 1995). Additionally, many other factors could also potentially be facilitators of aggression in sport. Table 1 summarizes the sources of influence on aggressive behaviors in team sports discussed in this section.

Multicausality

Most of the factors in Table 1 can be considered cues that can potentially trigger aggression under certain conditions or in combination with other variables (Bakker et al., 1995; Goldstein, 1983; Husman, 1980). Typically, an aggressive

Variable Type	Description
Intrapersonal	Arousal/emotions stemming from frustration
	Situational and generalized expectancies
	Perceptions and judgments of an opponent's action
	Aggressive cues (trivial) of individual significance
	Attitude toward aggression in sport generally
	Attitude toward aggression in their sport
Interpersonal	Frequency and severity of opponents' aggressive behavior
	Coaches' expectations that players be aggressive
	Coaches' instructions (explicit and implicit)
	Coaches' general behavior:
	- verbal, supportive/encouraging of aggression
	- nonverbal, supportive/encouraging of aggression
	Officials' bias towards one team
	Officials' incompetence:
	- type 1; miss an aggressive offense when it occurs
	- type 2; wrongly penalize legitimate behavior
	Officials' style:
	- authoritarian
	- relaxed
	Frequency and severity of teammates' aggression:
	- as a team (collective norms)
	- as individual players
	Reinforcement given to a player's aggression by teammates
Intergroup/Intragroup	Frequency of competition between teams
	Winning or losing team
	Visiting or home team
	League standing of teams
	Closeness of score
	Time gone in the game (Game time)
	Importance of game
	Criticalness of (within) game events
	Team norms/Deindividuation
Environmental	Home or away support
	Fans' abuse of players
	Fans' encouragement of aggression
	Size and density of crowd
	Fans' reaction to game events
	Heat
	Off-field issues

Table 1. Summary of sources of influence on aggressive behavior in sport

act will not be the result of only one causal event. Aggression is most likely a result of a combination of factors. It is likely that a number of factors interact or follow each other in order to bring about an occurrence of aggressive behavior. It is theorized that the more causal factors present, the greater the likelihood that an aggressive response will occur (Berkowitz, 1978). Also, the severity of an aggressive response may be a function of the amount and intensity of factors present. The sequence or combination of causal variables is not easily specified, and factors may operate simultaneously.

Measurements and Observation of Behaviors

To account for the behaviors of athletes when they occur (i.e., ecological validity), measurement of attitudes and opinions are required, along with reflections made by the athletes themselves, their coaches, their teammates, and the referees. Also, the "historical background" has to be taken into account, as it should be considered an important antecedent to the observed behaviors. We briefly reflect on these issues when we discuss aggressive behaviors.

Introspective Instrumentation

The most widely used self-report questionnaire to measure aggressive behavior in sport is the 50-item Athletic Aggression Inventory (BAAGI; Bredemeier, 1978). However, the accuracy of the BAAGI, which assesses instrumental and reactive aggression, has been called into question (Cox, 1990; LeUnes & Nation, 1986). Other tests, such as the Rosenzweig Picture-Frustration Study (Rosenzweig, 1950), the Team Norm Questionnaire (Shields et al., 1995), and the Aggressive Tendencies in Basketball Questionnaire (ATBQ; Duda, Olson, & Templin, 1991) have been developed for specific research purposes and have had limited application. The ATBQ assesses an individual's agreement with and reasoning about aggressive behaviors in basketball, specifically the perceived legitimacy of injurious acts (Duda, personal communication, September 25, 1996).

It is widely recognized that psychometric tests have inherent self-report bias and perennial problems with validity (Russell & Russell, 1984; Vokey & Russell, 1992). Worrell and Harris (1986) found that ice hockey players inaccurately perceived the amount of aggression they committed as measured by the BAAGI, when compared with objectively observed aggression. It should be stressed that, despite their continued use and their convenient nature, self-report, introspective measures alone have limited value in understanding sports aggression in real competitive settings. Psychometric tests are best applied in conjunction with more ecologically valid and objective measures (i.e., naturalistic observation).

Archival Data

The use of game information (i.e., penalties) and other match statistics, typically from past seasons and recorded by official scorers, has been a widely employed measure of aggression (Cox, 1990; Frank & Gilovich, 1988; Kelly & McCarthy, 1979; Russell & Drewry, 1976; Varca, 1980). Russell and Russell (1984), and in a replication, Vokey and Russell (1992) strongly supported selected sports penalties as a valid measure of aggression in sport. Noting the problems of construct and ecological validity with questionnaires and other measurement categories, such as projective tests and laboratory behavioral measures, they advocated the use of sports penalties as the most valid means of measuring aggression. However, they gave scant consideration to the alternative of observational analysis and neglected to rebuff any of the limitations of the archival method. Furthermore, the limitations of the method are evident in Russell and Russell's (1984) findings as to the determinants behind the aggressive penalties analyzed. The factor analysis approach they employed reduced 19 penalties to eight broad aggressive behavioral categories and offered no empirical evidence as to causation.

There are three main problems or restrictions with the archival approach. Not every aggressive behavior violates a sport's rules and is recorded as an infringement; not all penalties (even those distinguished as typically imposed for aggressive play) are due to aggressive behavior, and not all inappropriate acts of aggression are identified by officials (Bar-Eli & Tenenbaum, 1989; Mark et al., 1983).

In efforts to conduct more sophisticated studies based around archival data, attempts were made to distinguish between the types of rule infractions recorded as penalties in relation to aggression-based and nonaggressive infractions (Kelly & McCarthy, 1979; Russell, 1974; Russell & Drewry, 1976; Russell & Russell, 1984; Vokey & Russell, 1992). However, the classifications used had no theoretical basis, relied on experimenter discretion, and lacked empirical validation. In an effort to move the distinction between rule violations away from novice researchers to expert players, Widmeyer and Birch (1984) asked elite ice hockey players to differentiate between aggressive and non-aggressive penalties. In doing so, they were among the few researchers to operationalize a theoretically consistent definition of aggressive behavior (as distinct from nonaggressive behavior) and were the first to provide an empirical basis for establishing specific behaviors as aggressive.

McGuire et al. (1992) also followed this approach. Nevertheless, the limitation of measures of aggression based on data collection from official game reports and penalty records remains with this method. Widmeyer and Birch (1984) assumed that unnoticed aggressive acts and wrongly penalized acts were equally distributed across teams. However, because unpenalized behavior may be even more frequent than violations actually called (Bar-Eli & Tenenbaum, 1989), such an assumption is questionable. Also, the authors gave no consideration to the occurrence of aggressive behaviors that did not violate the rules of ice hockey.

Observational Methods

It has been recognized that to achieve more ecologically valid findings, sport psychology researches need to undertake more field studies (Cox, 1990). Although traditionally the least-used method, naturalistic observation is increasingly used today for research on aggression in sport (Bar-Eli & Tenenbaum, 1989; Cox, 1990; Harrell, 1980), most notably in applied settings.

The observation of behavior occurring in natural settings provides a valuable opportunity for researchers to better understand the complex dynamics of aggressive behavior in sport. Other research methods discussed have been of limited success in facilitating increased knowledge of such dynamics. Aggression remains best studied in real time and in the context in which it occurs. Practical constraints, such as the need for extensive training of observers, expense, and lengthy data analysis, have traditionally been the main barriers to observational research. Today, through the use of the computer and video technology, these logistic difficulties can be mostly overcome, and observational analysis can be used in a more sophisticated manner.

The use of a complementary questionnaire helps overcome the one inherent problem in studying aggression through observational methods, no matter how sophisticated the equipment used. That is, it is not always possible to be certain about the purpose (intent) behind an observed behavior. Making such a distinction can be difficult at times, when only overt behavioral acts are relied upon to determine intentionality and causality. For instance, with any given act of one player pushing another, observers can never be completely sure of the intent or determinants behind the behavior, especially if behavioral acts are observed independently of any meaningful contextual information.

With observational analysis, intentionality is essentially inferred. Experts—using repeated replay, following sport-specific behavioral typologies, and incorporating typical intention and severity of actions—make such inferences under rigorous research conditions. This approach is an advancement over the use of penalized behaviors (Russell & Russell, 1984; Widmeyer & Birch, 1984), in which officials (in the past) made similar inferences without the aid of repeated replays and were restricted by broad penalty groupings; inferences were retrospectively classified by researchers. Thus it is the case that on some occasions "true" intent, and thus the true nature of behavior (aggressive or not), may not be correctly established.

In the determination of causality, the use of observational analysis in conjunction with the incorporation of questionnaire data and players' and officials' comments while confronted by a video replay of behaviors of interest again has an advantage over previous methodologies. Self and other report information on causation can be used in association with observed antecedents to aggression.

Use of Experts

Experts have been used previously to assess the nature of aggressive-like behaviors (Bar-Eli & Tenenbaum, 1989; Teipel, Gerisch, & Busse, 1983; Widmeyer & Birch, 1984). Bar-Eli and Tenenbaum (1989) used experienced basketball players (who were also coaches) to observe behaviors that violated the rules and asked them to classify the behaviors as minor or major (essentially aggressive acts) violations. Widmeyer and Birch (1984) had elite ice hockey players differentiate between aggressive and nonaggressive penalties in ice hockey. Teipel et al. (1983) used ex-coaches and ex-players as a control group in their study comparing officials', players', and coaches' evaluations of fouls in soccer.

In these previous studies, the experts used were not directly involved in the behaviors under investigation. They were using their personal experience to infer the intention behind acts committed in general (Widmeyer & Birch,

1984) or by others (Bar-Eli & Tenenbaum, 1989; Teipel et al., 1983). A preferable method is to use experts involved in the observed behaviors of interest. Furthermore, the role of the experts can be expanded to include the following: categorization of behaviors (taxonomies for coding), questionnaire development, observation of behaviors, and inferences of causation.

Triangulation of Sources in Interpreting Behaviors

It is not our intention to describe in detail the procedures we have applied to study aggressive behaviors in basketball and ice hockey. However, we will briefly introduce the methodological plan to observe and account for the aggressive behaviors that occurred during the competitions we attended and filmed.

Development of Behavioral Typologies

This phase involved the development of behavioral typologies for the classification and coding of aggressive behavior. Aggressive-like behaviors in basketball and ice hockey were listed and categorized. This phase consisted of the following three stages:

Stage 1: Compilation of behaviors used in previous studies to measure aggression (or to differentiate aggression). Scanning of relevant literature was carried out on aggression and documented behaviors used in previous research on ice hockey and basketball as measures of aggression.

Stage 2: Experts' selection of aggressive behaviors. After being briefed about the definition of aggression, the experts individually noted behaviors that they considered to be aggressive in nature from their sport. Behaviors identified by experts that were not collated in Stage 1 were added to the list.

Stage 3: Classification of behaviors: Development of taxonomies of behavior. The respective aggressive-like basketball and ice hockey behaviors derived were classified based on theoretical principles and experts' comments according to three dimensions:

1. Physical or nonphysical behavior.
2. Assertive or aggressive act based on the intent typically associated with such behavior.
3. Rating of typical severity of each behavioral type, on a continuum from assertive acts to very violent acts.

Behaviors common to both sports were considered for each sport separately. Thus, behaviors were classified according to the sport context.

The resulting taxonomies of behavior for each sport are presented in Tables 2 and 3. Behavioral types were grouped according to the above dimensions. Descriptions of what each behavior constitutes and the penalty typically imposed by officials for the occurrence of each behavioral type during a game are also provided in the tables. It was found that behaviors vary in their specificity. It can be seen that some more general behaviors encompass others. For example, "fighting" in ice hockey is a broad category that can include pushing and kicking, whereas "assaulting" in basketball can include grabbing and shoulder butting.

Behavior	Description	Penalty Typically Imposed by Official
Physical Behaviors		
Nonaggressive		
Interference	When a player impedes the goalkeeper or a player not in possession of the puck. Also, if a player deliberately knocks the stick from a player's hand or impedes a player who has lost his stick from retrieving it.	A minor penalty. Gross misconduct penalty if a player on the bench interferes.
Holding	When a player impedes (or seeks to) a player by "holding" that player in any way, including grabbing a player's stick.	A minor penalty.
Hooking	When a player impedes (or seeks to) a player by using the stick to "hook" them.	A minor penalty. Major penalty if injury results.
Tripping	When a player places his stick, foot, arm, knee, hand, elbow, in such a manner that it causes a player to "trip" or fall.	A minor penalty. Exception to this is when puck carrier is in goal scoring position (in the attacking zone with only the goalkeeper to beat) and is tripped from behind, then a penalty shot is awarded.

Table 2. Taxonomy of ice hockey behaviors used for
observational coding of aggression

Behavior	Description	Penalty Typically Imposed by Official
Physical Behaviors		
Aggressive		
Butt-ending	When a player pokes a player with the point ("butt" end) of the stick.	A minor penalty. Major penalty if injury results or if against goalkeeper within his crease.
Clipping	When a player slides into a puck carrier's path so that he loses possession.	A minor penalty. Major penalty if injury results.
Cross-checking	When a player uses the stick with both hands to block across the upper body of a player (no part of the stick is on the ground).	A minor penalty. Major penalty if injury results, or if against goalkeeper within his crease.
High Sticking	When a player contacts a player with a stick carried above shoulder height (see cross-checking).	A minor penalty.
Shoulder Butting	When a player deliberately drives his shoulder into a player.	A minor penalty.
Pushing	When a player deliberately pushes or shoves a player.	A minor penalty. Major penalty if injury results.
Charging	When a player checks (or hits) a player with excessive force, while taking more than two steps in that player's direction.	A minor penalty. Major penalty if injury results or if charge from behind or against goalkeeper within his crease.
Elbowing	When a player fouls a player by using his or her elbow.	A minor penalty. Major penalty if injury results.
Kneeing	When a player fouls a player by using his or her knee.	A minor penalty. Major penalty if injury results.
Roughing	Use of excessive force ("roughness") in any game situation.	A major penalty.
Spitting	When a player spits at (or in the direction of) a player.	A misconduct penalty.

Table 2. Taxonomy of ice hockey behaviors used for observational coding of aggression

Behavior	Description	Penalty Typically Imposed by Official
Physical Behaviors		
Aggressive		
Boarding	When a player checks (or hits) a player in such a manner that the player is thrown into the boards violently.	A major penalty.
Grabbing	When a player strongly impedes the progress of a player or pulls the player toward him or her by clutching or grabbing the player or the player's face mask.	A major penalty.
Slashing	When a player impedes (or seeks to) a player by "slashing" him/her with the stick.	A major penalty.
Spearing	When a player uses the stick to poke or "spear" a player (see butt-ending).	Typically a minor penalty is imposed. Major penalty if injury results or if against goalkeeper within his crease.
Checking from behind	When a player pushes, body checks, or hits a player from behind in any manner, or knocks a player from behind into the boards in such a way that the player is unable to protect himself or herself.	A major penalty.
Violent		
Fighting	There are three general categories of behavior: a) Starting a fight (instigating) by emitting aggressive violent behavior, b) Fighting back with aggressive or violent behavior, and c) Continuing to fight back.	For 'b' a major penalty; for 'a' & 'c', match penalties.

Table 2. Taxonomy of ice hockey behaviors used for observational coding of aggression

Behavior	Description	Penalty Typically Imposed by Official
Physical Behaviors		
Violent		
	Within these, there are differing types of fighting:	
Stick Swinging Fist Fighting	d) Stick use (e.g., stick swinging). e) Fist fighting (i.e., punching, gloves and helmet taken off, stick down). f) Brawling, involving a number of players (ranging from two or three players to bench-clearing) and constituting a possible range of aggressive and violent behavior.	Either major or match penalties.
Kicking	g) When a player deliberately kicks a player.	A match penalty.
Headbutting	h) When a player deliberately strikes a player with his or her head.	A match penalty.
Nonphysical Behaviors		
Aggressive to Violent		
Self-abuse Abuse a player	There are three general categories of behavior, ranging in severity from verbal abuse: a) Towards oneself, b) Towards another player, and c) Towards an official (severe verbal negatives).	'a' is not penalized; for 'b' a misconduct penalty is imposed; for 'c' a gross misconduct penalty.
Negative verbalisation to officials	Within these, there are differing types of behavior:	As above
Swearing	d) Comments of a questioning nature, e) Swearing, and f) Insulting (the most severe verbal behavior; especially when toward an official.	

Table 2. Taxonomy of ice hockey behaviors used for observational coding of aggression

Behavior	Description	Penalty Typically Imposed by Official
Physical Behaviors		
Nonaggressive		
Obstruction	When a player blocks or impedes (or seeks to) the progress of another player.	A personal foul.
Minor Contact	Whenever a player makes minor and unintentional contact with another player.	Not penalized.
Charging	When a player moves in a forceful manner towards another player's body.	Not penalized. If contact with a player, a personal foul is called unless the player touched obstructs player moving or makes little effort to play ball.
Pushing	When a player pushes another player without severe intent.	Not penalized.
Aggressive		
Rear Guarding	When a player has contact with another player while guarding him or her from the rear.	A personal foul.
Hand Checking	When a player uses hand contact to control the movement of another player.	A personal foul.
Swinging Arm	When a player swings his or her arm or arms around or in the direction of another player.	A personal foul.
Holding	When a player intentionally impedes (or seeks to) or prevents another player from moving by grab-bing/clutching that player in any way.	A personal foul.
Assaulting	A general category of behavior. When a player has forceful physical contact with another player without attempting to get the ball (including off-the-ball play).	A personal foul.

Table 3. Taxonomy of basketball behaviors used for observational coding of aggression

Behavior	Description	Penalty Typically Imposed by Official
Physical Behaviors		
Aggressive		
Shoulder Butting	When a player knocks or butts a player with his or her shoulder.	A personal foul.
Grabbing	When a player strongly "grabs" or wrestles with another player with the intention of impeding or holding back the player. A forceful holding.	A personal foul.
Slapping	When a player deliberately strikes another player or him- or herself using an open hand.	If minor or against oneself, a personal foul is called. If more severe, an intentional foul is called.
Shoving	When a player strongly and deliberately pushes another player. A severe push.	A personal foul.
Elbowing	When a player fouls another player by using his or her elbow.	A personal foul.
Tripping	When a player places a foot, leg, or body in such a manner that it causes another player to trip or fall.	A personal foul.
Throwing the Ball Away	When a player intentionally throws the ball out of the court or out of the reach of the team to take possession of it.	A technical foul.
Spitting	When a player spits at (or in the direction of) another player.	A technical foul.
Violent		
Throwing the Ball	When a player deliberately throws the ball at another player, or in severe cases an official.	An intentional foul.
Punching	When a player deliberately strikes another player with a closed fist.	An intentional foul.

Table 3. Taxonomy of basketball behaviors used for observational coding of aggression

Behavior	Description	Penalty Typically Imposed by Official
Physical Behaviors		
Violent		
Kicking	When a player intentionally kicks another player.	An intentional foul.
Nonphysical Behaviors		
Nonaggressive		
Negative Comments	When a player questions or expresses negative comments in regard to an official's or a player's action, or criticizes his or her own play.	Not penalized.
Pacing Around	When a player walks around the court in a frustrated or angry manner (includes slapping one's hand or shaking one's head in disgust, etc).	Not penalized.
Aggressive		
Insulting	Severe negative comments, or when players verbally abuse (can include swearing) in order of severity.	Not penalized.
Self-abuse	a) Themselves b) Member/s of the crowd	'a' and 'b' are not penalized.
Abuse of player	c) Another player	'c' depends on severity, technical foul if major.
Abuse of official	d) An official Also: e) Coach disrespectfully or aggressively addresses officials, or aggressively addresses his players or opponents.	for 'd' a technical foul is usually called. If minor, not penalized; if moderate typically a technical foul is called. If severe or frequent coach may be banned from court vicinity.

Table 3. Taxonomy of basketball behaviors used for observational coding of aggression

Introspective Measures and Filming

This phase involved the administration of questionnaires to players and officials (Stage 1) and the filming of the selected basketball and ice hockey games (Stage 2).

Stage 1: Administration of questionnaires. At a training session a few days prior to the first basketball game and the second ice hockey game to be filmed, players were given the respective ice hockey or basketball version of the questionnaire to complete. Officials (experts) were given their associated questionnaire to complete at their convenience.

Stage 2: Filming of games. Over a 2-week period, four selected fixtures were filmed. For each game, two cameras were used: One camera was directed to the play; the other on the court/rinkside behavior of coaches and substitutes. In addition, microphones were placed on the officials and on the sidelines to pick up comments from the bench and the crowd.

Interpretation of Causation, Intention, and Severity of Behaviors

This phase involved the experts' and the experimenter's classification, consideration of causation, and rating of aggressive-like behavior from the obtained video footage (Stage 1), the coding of aggressive behaviors (Stage 2), and the consideration of intentions of players exhibiting behaviors (Stage 3).

Stage 1: Classification, consideration of causation, and rating of aggressive-like behaviors. The experimenter and each expert individually and the experimenter viewed the footage of either the two recorded basketball or the two recorded ice hockey games. On the second viewing, experts in conjunction with the experimenter were instructed to (a) note each occurrence of a forceful act as either assertive or aggressive behavior (based on their judged intent and observed severity of the acts), (b) whenever possible, categorize each behavior exhibited in accordance with the behavioral taxonomies developed in the first phase of the study (e.g., code each individual behavior as a push, kick, or a punch), (c) rate each behavior (given its intention and the context it occurred) in terms of severity, from 1 (least severe) to 5 (most severe), and (d) note what they thought the cause or causes were of each aggressive act. (To avoid leading questions, open responses were used. Experts expressed causation in their own terms.)

Behaviors were always classified according to the game context. It was considered that similar behaviors might have had different intent and force in different occasions and situations. For example, in one circumstance a player directing comments towards another player was judged to have the intention of distracting the other player from the game, whereas in another situation, his intent was judged to be to upset (psychologically harm) the other player. Similarly, checking in ice hockey and the use of elbows in basketball were considered nonaggressive behavior whenever these behaviors were judged to be driven by the goal to effect good play and not by the intent to injure. In contrast, whenever it was considered that excessive force occurred in carrying out the behavior, or that the intent was to inflict harm, then acts were recorded as being aggressive.

The severity ratings used were standard across behavior types. That is, a rating of "3" for a push referred to the overall severity of the behavior in general across all aggressive behaviors, not the degree of severity in comparison to other pushes. Within behavioral type, comparisons could also be made. A relatively severe push rated as a "3," for example, might have been of the same severity as a punch rated as a "3," but such a punch could be considered a relatively nonsevere punch, as behaviors of that type were usually rated as "4" or "5."

Experts involved (officiating) in the games under investigation and thus involved in behaviors coded as aggressive were specifically asked what they were thinking at the time the behaviors of interest occurred (i.e., What were their attitudes and perceptions?). They were also asked why they did or did not penalize the aggressive acts.

The experts' responses were recorded. The combined information was analyzed into listings of times and descriptions of the recorded behavioral act in preparation for formal computer (CAMERA) coding (Stage 2). The focus was on combining the experts' knowledge with the experimenter's objective determination of aggression in order to create the most accurate behavior classifications.

Stage 2: Computerized coding of aggressive behaviors. When a computerized system is used, the coding of the prerecorded aggressive behaviors (Stage 1) in a consistent and systematic manner is taking place. Severity ratings of acts and the details of the players committing them, along with causal inferences, were recorded on the computer outputs of the coded behavior.

Stage 3: Consideration of intentions of players' emitting behaviors. Some of the players participating in the filmed games and emitting the behavior coded as aggressive replayed the acts they were involved in and were asked what they were thinking at the time (i.e., What were their attitudes and their intentions?). Information from the players' responses to relevant questionnaire items was used to aid this stage. The information derived at this stage was collated in conjunction with the outputs from the previous stage.

Making Inferences and Conclusions

This phase involved examination of causation. Preceding and subsequent game events were coded, and variables reported in the literature were considered in relation to the most severe aggressive behavior, and the observational analysis was made by combining data sources to produce time-behavior (including attitudes) analysis forms.

Stage 1: Coding of game antecedents to the most severe aggressive acts and events following these acts. The computerized system was used to code relevant game events immediately preceding and immediately following the most severe aggressive acts (mostly involving violent behavior) in each of the filmed games. The experts in the previous stage of the study provided the temporally related events or behaviors that were systematically coded.

Up to four minutes of footage on both before and after the most severe aggressive act from each game were analyzed. Exact starting and stopping points depended on events of interest. Details of the player(s) committing the behavior and those who were the targets of the behavior were recorded on the computer output of the coded behavior, along with game score and any other corresponding factual information of relevance. Additionally, potential source variables, factors found in the literature to be related to aggression or hypothesized to be associated with aggression, were monitored. Indications for the influence of all such variables were systematically checked for and noted whenever possible evidence was found.

Stage 2: Collation of all observed behavioral acts and recorded factors of influence. Incorporation of all relevant information in the study into documented time-behavior paths was carried out.

Integration of Sources of Evidence

Once the attitudes towards aggression were measured, the "competitive histories" between the teamswere documented, the games filmed, and the players', coaches', and referees' reflections were recorded. The data should be integrated and then interpreted. We do not intend to present all the data analyses in this chapter, as the aim here is to introduce the methodological framework of studying behaviors of players in team sports. However, several important examples are introduced.

To examine ice hockey and basketball players' attitudes toward aggressive acts, six scenarios of aggression, ranging from mild to severe, were given to them in each of their respective sports. The summary of their collective responses is presented in Table 4. It can be observed from the Table that the aggressive tendencies of both the basketball and ice hockey players varied in line with the scenario presented to them. Also, it can be seen that the ice hockey players exhibited greater approval of aggressive acts than did basketball players. This is in line with the nature and practices of the two games.

Abbreviated Scenario	Ice Hockey		Basketball		Sports Combined	
	M	SD	M	SD	M	SD
Give a dirty look to an opponent	1.91	0.74	2.06	0.57	1.96	0.68
Muscle out an opponent	2.16	1.35	1.74	0.59	2.02	1.15
Punch an opponent	3.91	0.85	3.74	1.25	3.85	0.96
Cause an opponent's concussion	3.12	1.18	3.86	0.77	3.35	1.11
Cause tearing an opponent's ligaments	3.96	1.12	4.60	0.72	4.17	1.03
Permanently disable an opponent	3.93	1.11	4.34	0.89	4.07	1.04

Note: Lower ratings indicate greater approval with the aggressive scenario portrayed.

Table 4. Table of means and SDs for scenarios of ice hockey, basketball, and sports combine across situations

In the study of the history of aggressive acts between the teams, only 17% of the basketball players reported that a teammate had had a previous aggressive encounter with a member or members of the opposition, whereas 75% of ice hockey players reported so. However, on the individual level, a higher percentage of basketball players (50%) reported that they personally had had a previous aggressive encounter with a member of the opposition team compared to ice hockey players (38%). All basketball players responded that the upcoming game to be filmed was important, whereas just under half (47%) of the ice hockey players so responded.

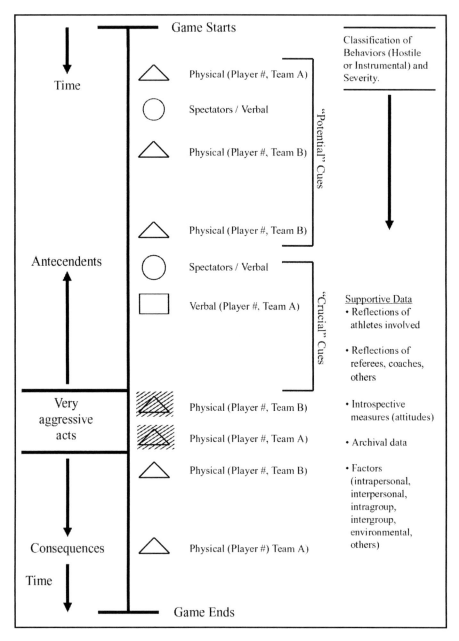

Figure 2. Integrating sources of evidence in team competitions and derivation of casualty

It was evident from the basketball players' open responses that the teams involved in the first basketball game were current and/or traditional "rivals," and that players from both teams expected (in all but one case) their opponents to be very aggressive. There was a notable difference in the responses of the two ice hockey teams in regard to why their second game was important. Only four ice hockey players (25%) did not expect their opponents to be aggressive (including two who were uncertain). The home team, which, according to league records, had lost eight consecutive games to the away team, cited "not having beaten" their opponents and providing an "indication of their improvement" as reasons, whereas the successful away team players cited the cliché "every game is important" as the only reason.

The questionnaire responses of the four officials (two from each sport) were also utilized. Both basketball officials (the involved one and the independent one) expected the game of interest to be aggressive, and both were familiar with particular players they considered aggressive and whom they would typically "keep their eye on." Both basketball officials also indicated that aggressive play generally has a place in sport, as long as it is within game rules. In comparison, both ice hockey officials knew of numerous previous aggressive encounters between players. The involved ice hockey official was officiating his 17th and 18th games involving one or both of the two teams this current season. He felt that aggressive play generally has a place in sport as long as it is "within game rules" or is "controlled aggression" rather than "naked aggression."

The analysis of the filmed games revealed that a majority of the total aggressive acts coded were physical in nature, 107 versus 60 nonphysical. Basketball had 41 acts of physical aggression and 25 of nonphysical aggression. The totals for ice hockey were 66 and 35, respectively. For both sports, all acts directed to officials were oral in nature.

The main concerns for the observational data on events prior and subsequent to the most severe aggressive acts found in the games were coded based on experts' advice. This information was analyzed in conjunction with questionnaire responses, other recorded comments from players and officials, and additional documented game-related information and included consideration of a range of causal variables identified in the literature (e.g., Anshel, 1994). Time-behavior tables developed around the tracing of events prior to and following the occurrence of the severe aggressive acts of interest were established. In each case, reference was made to the players involved in the aggressive behaviors. Behaviors were classified as either hostile or instrumental, and their severity ratings were established; nonobservable data of relevance (framed whenever appropriate in terms of causal factors) were also added. The integrated sources of evidence are shown in Figure 2.

The application of such a methodology to the study of aggressive behaviors in ice hockey and basketball revealed that antecedents to aggressive acts in ice hockey were: other physically aggressive acts, forceful play, little time left, close score, anger and negative attitudes toward the target of aggression, and sometimes a player's having a known history of aggression. The consequences were further aggressive acts, ongoing verbal abuse, change in teammates' support, and penalties by the referees. In basketball, aggressive acts were preceded by other physical acts of less severity, loss of possession/missed shots, string of points by one team, close score, preexisting grudges between players involved in the act, and officials' lack of appropriate responses. The consequences were crowd reaction, continual scoring of more points by the team that was the target of aggression rather than by the aggressive team, teammates/crowd support, and officials' correctly penalizing judged instigator.

Such information, when integrated with players' reflection, indicated that the causes of aggression in sport cannot be sufficiently accounted for by only one of the three theories. Each of these theories accounts for some of the behaviors. An integrated theory should be established that takes into account the uniqueness of team sports and all the factors that potentially may result in aggressive and assertive behaviors.

We recommend that the study of behaviors in team sport follow the methodological concept presented here. Variations may be necessary, depending on the aims of the study and other factors that may limit or extend the scope of the investigation. However, a departure from the concept should consider both practical and theoretical grounds.

References

Anshel, M. H. (1994). *Sport psychology: From theory to practice.* Scottsdate, AZ: Gorsuch.

Bakker, F. C., Whiting, H. T., & Van der Brug, H. (1995). *Sport psychology: Concepts and applications.* Chichester, UK: Wiley.

Bandura, A. (1979). The social learning perspective: Mechanisms of aggression. In H. Toch (Ed.), *Psychology of crime and criminal justice* (pp. 198-236). New York: Holt Rinehart and Winston.

Bar-Eli, M., & Tenenbaum, G. (1989). Observations of behavioral violations as crisis indicators in competition. *The Sport Psychologist, 3,* 237-244.

Berkowitz, L. (1978). Whatever happened to the frustration-aggression hypothesis? *American Behavioral Scientist, 21,* 691-708.

Bredemeier, B. J. (1978). The assessment of reactive and instrumental athletic aggression. In E. Geron (Ed.), *Proceedings of the International Symposium on Psychological Assessment.* Netanya, Israel: Wingate Institute.

Bredemeier, B. J. (1985). Moral reasoning and the perceived legitimacy of intentionally injurious sports acts. *Journal of Sport Psychology, 7,* 110-124.

Chalmers, A. F. (1982). *What is this thing called science?* Brisbane, Australia: University of Queensland Press.

Connelly, D. (1988). Increasing intensity of play of nonassertive athletes. *The Sport Psychologist, 2,* 255-265.

Courneya, K. S., & Carron, A. V. (1992). The home advantage in sport competitions: A literature review. *Journal of Sport and Exercise Psychology, 14,* 13-27.

Cox, R. (1990). *Sport psychology: Concepts and applications.* Dubuque, IA:WCB.

Dollard, J., Miller, N., Doob, I., Mourer, O. H., & Sears, R. R. (1939). *Frustration and aggression.* New Haven, CT: Yale University Press.

Duda, J., Olson, K., & Templin, T. (1991). The relationship of task and ego orientation to sportsmanship attitudes and the perceived legitimacy of injurious acts. *Research Quarterly for Exercise and Sport, 62,* 79-86.

Frank, M. G., & Gilovich, T. (1988). The dark side of self and social perception: Black uniforms and aggression in professional sports. *Journal of Personality and Social Psychology, 54,* 74-85.

Gelso, C., & Mandracchia, C. (1983). Aggressiveness and sexual habits regarding the players of an amateur football team. *Journal of Andrology, 4,* 53-54.

Goldstein, J. H. (1983). (Ed.). *Sports violence.* New York: Springer-Verlag.

Harrell, W. A. (1980). Aggression by high school basketball players: An observational study of the effects of opponents' aggression and frustration inducing factors. *International Journal of Sport Psychology, 11,* 190-298.

Husman, B. (1980). Aggression: An historical perspective. In W. F. Straub (Ed.), *Sport psychology: An analysis of athlete behavior* (pp. 182-186). Ithaca, NY: Mouvement.

Husman, B., & Silva, J. M., III. (1984). Aggression in sport: definitional and theoretical considerations. In J. M. Silva & R. S. Weinberg (Eds.), *Psychological foundations of sport* (pp. 246-260). Champaign, IL: Human Kinetics.

Kelly, B. R., & McCarthy, J. F. (1979). Personality dimensions of aggression and its relationship to time and place of action in ice hockey. *Human Relations, 32,* 219-225

LeFebrve, L. M., & Passer, M. W. (1974). The effects of game location and importance on aggression in team sport. *International Journal of Sport Psychology, 12,* 102-110.

Leith, L. M. (1982). The role of competition in the elicitation of aggression in sport. *Journal of Sport Behavior, 5,* 168-174.

LeUnes, A. D., & Nation, J. R. (1989). *Sport psychology: An introduction.* Chicago: Nelson Hall.

Luxbacher, J. A. (1986). Violence in sports: An examination of the theories of aggression and how the coach can influence the degree of violence displayed in sport. *Coaching Review, 9,* 14-17.

Mark, M. M., Bryant, F. B., & Lehman, D. R. (1983). Perceived injustice and sports violence. In J. H. Goldstein (Ed.), *Sports violence* (pp. 83-109). New York: Springer-Verlag.

Martin, L. A. (1976). Effects of competition upon the aggressive responses of college basketball players and wrestlers. *Research Quarterly, 47,* 338-393.

McGuire, E. J., Courneya, K. S., Widmeyer, W. N., & Carron, A. V. (1992). Aggression as a potential mediator of the home advantage in professional ice hockey. *Journal of Sport and Exercise Psychology, 14,* 148-158.

Pfister, R. (1982). Aggression and sports practice: Testing the cathartic value of sport. *Bulletin de Psychologie (French), 35,* 88-100.

Reifman, A. S., Larrick, R. P., & Fein, S. (1991). Temper and temperature on the diamond: The heat-aggression relationship in major league baseball. *Personality and Social Psychology Bulletin, 17,* 580-585.

Rosenzweig, S. (1950). *Revised scoring manual for the Rosenzweig Picture-Frustration Study, form for adults.* St. Louis, MO: Author.

Russell, G. W. (1974). Machiavellianism, locus of control, aggression, performance and precautionary behavior in ice hockey. *Human Relations, 27,* 825-837.

Russell, G. W. (1981a). Conservatism, birth order, leadership, and the aggression of Canadian ice hockey players. *Perceptual and Motor Skills, 53,* 3-7.

Russell, G. W. (1981b). Spectator moods at an aggressive sports event. *Journal of Sport Psychology, 3,* 217-227.

Russell, G. W., & Drewry, B. R. (1976). Crowd size and competitive aspects of aggression in ice hockey: An archival study. *Human Relations, 29,* 723-735.

Russell, G. W., & Russell, A. M. (1984). Sports penalties: An alternative means of measuring aggression. *Social Behavior and Personality, 12,* 69-74.

Schneider, J., & Eitzen, D. (1986). The structure of sport and participant violence. In R. Lapchick (Ed.), *Fractured focus: Sport as a reflection of society* (pp. 228-242). Lexington, MS: D.C. Heath.

Shields, D. L., Bredemeier, B. J., Gardner, D. E., & Bostrom, A. (1995). Leadership, cohesion, and team norms regarding cheating and aggression. *Sociology of Sport Journal, 12,* 324-336.

Silva, J. M., III. (1980). Understanding aggressive behavior and its effects upon athletic performance. In W. F. Straub (Ed.), *Sport psychology: An analysis of athlete behavior* (pp. 179-186). Ithaca, NY: Mouvement.

Smith, M .D. (1980). Violence in hockey. In W. F. Straub (Ed.), *Sport psychology: An analysis of athlete behavior* (pp. 187-192). Ithaca, NY: Mouvement.

Smith, M. D. (1982). Social determinants of violence in hockey: A review. In R. Magill, M. Ash, & F. Smoll (Eds.), *Children in sport* (pp. 301-313). Champaign, IL: Human Kinetics.

Teipel, D., Gerisch, G., & Busse, M. (1983). Evaluation of aggressive behavior in football. *International Journal of Sport Psychology, 14,* 228-242.

Thirer, J. (1993). Aggression. In R. Singer, M. Murphy, & K. L. Tennant (Eds.), *Handbook of research on sport psychology* (pp. 365-378). New York: MacMillan.

Thirer, J., & Rampey, M. S. (1979). Effects of abusive spectators' behavior on performance of home and visiting intercollegiate basketball teams. *Perceptual and Motor Skills, 48,* 1047-1053.

Varca, P. (1980). An analysis of home and away game performance of male college basketball teams. *Journal of Sport Psychology, 2,* 246-257.

Vaz, E. W. (1977). Institutionalised rule violation in professional ice hockey: Perspectives and control systems. *Journal of the Canadian Association of Health, Physical Education and Recreation, 43,* 6-16.

Vokey, J. R., & Russell, G. W. (1992). On penalties as measures of aggression. *Social Behavior and Personality, 20,* 219-226.

Widmeyer, W. N., & Birch, J. S. (1984). Aggression in professional ice hockey: A strategy for success or a reaction to failure? *The Journal of Psychology, 117,* 77-84.

Widmeyer, W. N., & McGuire, E. J. (1997). Frequency of competition and aggression in professional ice hockey. *International Journal of Sport Psychology, 28,* 57-66.

Worrell, G. L., & Harris, D. V. (1986). The relationship of perceived and observed aggression of ice hockey players. *International Journal of Sport Psychology, 17,* 34-40.

CHAPTER 3

Ethical Issues in Team Sports

Richard D. Gordin

Abstract

This chapter contains a brief overview of common ethical concerns to be considered when one works with team sports. The first part of the chapter deals with the ethical guidelines established by both the Association for the Advancement of Applied Sport Psychology (AAASP) and the American Psychological Association (APA). The chapter also contains several anecdotes from the author's 25-year practice as an applied sport psychologist. The chapter concludes with several recommendations for the sport psychology consultant who works with team sports.

Every legitimate sport psychology organization around the world operates by a set of ethical principles and a code of conduct. In the United States, the American Psychological Association (APA) code, the Ethical Principles of Psychologists and Code of Conduct (American Psychological Association, 1992) is the appropriate standard to follow. Also, the Association for the Advancement of Applied Sport Psychology (AAASP) has adopted this set of ethical principles, with a few modifications, as advocated by the APA code (Etzel & Whelan, 1995; Meyers, 1995). In the United States there are two organizations that oversee the field of sport psychology: Division 47 of the APA, which represents more of the clinical side of the field, and the AAASP, which is more interested in the applied aspect of sport psychology. Petitpas, Brewer, Rivera, and Van Raalte (1994) conducted a survey of AAASP members to ascertain and obtain preliminary data on ethical beliefs and behavior practices of applied sport psychologists. They noted few differences as a function of gender, professional training, or academic discipline. However, results of open-ended questions indicated that most of the questionable ethical practices cited by respondents to the survey violated APA guidelines in some fashion. These findings provided support that AAASP needed to adopt the APA ethical guidelines and also institute training in ethics to the applied sport psychologists. In this chapter it is my intent to cover these principles and to illustrate various case examples of how these principles work in the real world and with team sports.

I have been a practicing sport psychology consultant for over 25 years, and my unique perspective will be the primary viewpoint of this chapter. After reading this chapter, each of you should be prompted to assess your own ethics and values. After all, each individual interprets and makes his or her own operational principles and ethics. In effect, we police ourselves.

Preamble

Sport psychologists fulfill many roles based upon their professional training and expertise. Professionals work diligently to develop a body of professional literature and knowledge based upon good science. Sport psychologists respect the freedom of academic inquiry and individual expression in the practice of sport psychology, whether it is in sport or exercise psychology settings. The statement adopted by the AAASP provides a set of principles designed to protect clients and establish good practice habits. A code of conduct does not insure competency. It is designed to provide an overview of acceptable practice procedures. AAASP members protect and respect human rights and civil rights, and do not knowingly discriminate unfairly. Members also encourage ethical behavior in the profession among members, students, and supervisees. All principles are followed with each member's personal value and culture and experience embedded in the practice and interpretation of these guidelines (paraphrased from Meyers, 1995).

This preamble serves a purpose for all sport psychology consultants. We must be able to act proactively and not reactively to potentially harmful situations. Our profession comprises individuals with a variety of training experiences. This preamble to a set of ethical guidelines is an attempt to level the field for conduct issues.

General Principles

There are six general principles to adhere to in terms of ethics and conduct in this field: Competence, integrity, professional and scientific responsibility, respect for people's rights and dignity, concern for others' welfare, and social responsibility.

Principle A: Competence

Psychologists strive to maintain high standards of competence in their work. They recognize the boundaries of their particular competency. They provide only services that they are qualified to provide based upon adequate training and certification. Practitioners also maintain an updated survey of the scientific evidence of information that is relevant to what they do. Ongoing education remains a must. They also are cognizant of the competencies required to serve a broad constituency of clients (paraphrased from Meyers, 1995).

The origins of the field of sport psychology are imbedded in sport science. Many of the early practitioners were trained in this discipline. It is therefore essential for all to become familiar with ethical dilemmas within psychology. However, the diversity of training experiences is beginning to meld sport science with psychology for the new sport psychology professionals. It is essential for all to be familiar with both fields. Likewise, if one has not experienced the world of sport from inside the locker room, it is possible for some grievous errors to occur in the practice of good sport psychology. If a clinical psychologist, for instance, blindly applies to sport the techniques that have been developed primarily for the clinical setting, it is possible for harm to occur. The typical solutions to clinical issues often do not fit in the sporting environment. The classic, yet absurd, example is that of a baseball player in a hitting slump. The clinical sport psychologist approaches the situation from a medical model and hypothesizes that there is some neurosis driving the slump. Someone within the organization suggests that the hitter seek the help of an ophthalmologist, and it is determined that a prescription change is all that is needed. We must be careful to ask the correct questions prior to delving into treatment. Likewise, athletes do not generally respond well to the "shrink" image of the provider. That is not to say that an athlete is immune to psychological problems. After all, athletes are ordinary people performing extraordinary physical feats. A sport psychologist trained in traditional sport science must possess the ability to distinguish true need for intervention for personal problems and learn to refer appropriately when necessary. Personal bias must also be recognized and adapted to practice. If, for instance, a sport psychology consultant brings the bias of prior experience with poor coaching into the consulting relationship, then a poor initial relationship with the coach might impede progress with the athlete.

The coach-athlete relationship is sacred in sport. If the sport psychologist places himself or herself between the coach and athlete, then failure will occur. The consultant will be dismissed and the athlete will lose out. Moreover, the consultant trained in sport science must recognize his or her lack of training in more clinically related procedures and refrain from experimenting with these procedures. This environment is delicate and does not lend itself to experimentation for the sake of training. I have found it invaluable over the years to have a group of colleagues with whom I can share my concerns and gather a professional consultation concerning my biases. I would encourage all who consult to develop a peer group that will serve this very purpose.

One of the controversial issues within sport psychology is psychological assessment. First of all, let me state my bias concerning this issue. I have used and continue to use psychological assessment over the past 25 years. I will follow the lead of Henschen (1997), who has argued that the question should not be whether testing should be used but rather who should test and under what guidelines. The training of all future and current sport psychology consultants should include psychological assessment. In our field, this has been a bitter dispute. I also believe that all sport psychology professionals use assessment in one way or another (i.e., subjective or objective). Psychological testing is not a panacea or an end in itself; rather it is a skill to be used to help athletes. It is unfortunate that the skill of psychological testing has been denigrated in our profession. If one is merely trying to obtain information that will aid in helping the athlete, then such testing is more than useful. One might argue that the APA's guidelines are the only appropriate guidelines to follow when administering tests. However, I believe that additional considerations are warranted. I would advocate the following guidelines in utilizing tests in sport psychology:

1. The individual being tested has the right to know why he or she is being tested and how the information will be used (with whom test results will be discussed and what will be discussed).

2. The athlete has the right to know the conclusions based upon test results. The sport psychologist has the responsibility to communicate the results in a way that is appropriate and understandable to the athlete. The use of professional and clinical jargon should be avoided.

3. The reports are given only to people who are able to interpret them and with the expressed permission of the test taker (athlete). Confidentiality must always be respected.

4. The tester must possess the appropriate training in administering and evaluating tests.

5. The sport psychologist should always administer the test face-to-face

and explain beforehand why the tests are given and with whom the results will be shared.

6. The testing results should always be triangulated and substantiated with the athlete. Observations and incongruencies should be resolved (Nideffer, 1981).

Psychological assessment is only one tool to use to gather pertinent information about athletes. Attending training sessions, observing competitive situations, and conducting personal interviews are also necessary and desirable actions before making decisions about interventions. If one follows the rudimentary professional guidelines mentioned, then one possesses a valuable tool to help the client. An illustration will perhaps demonstrate the concept of abuse of competence issues. I was once working with a prominent professional on the PGA Tour and had traveled to the U.S. Open to observe his play. At this point in our relationship, we had been working approximately two years together. Upon arrival the athlete was rather distraught at the idea that he had "flunked" a psychological test. He had been approached to take a psychological test by a sport psychologist. He showed me the test results that were scored and left in his locker by the psychologist. A "psychological profile" disclosed that he had a lower than average profile on several subscales of the test when compared with the average profile of excellent players. I had to interpret the results so that he understood the measurement error and the problems with averaging psychological data, and I reassured him that he was ready to play. The testing procedures were unethical and potentially very harmful on the part of the sport psychologist. This psychologist either did not understand the ethical competence issues of psychological testing or was ignorant of the existing guidelines. Information pertaining to psychological testing should always be presented face-to-face with the client in terms understandable to the athlete. Also, when information is shared, it should cause no harm. In addition, an athlete should not be tested before asking if he or she is in an ongoing relationship with another sport psychologist.

Another area of concern is the competence issues within team sports. An applied sport psychologist usually deals with team dynamics, group dynamics, conflict resolution, team motivation issues, general counseling issues, and assessment. Clinical sport psychologists generally deal with clinical issues of individual athletes that are affecting team performance and assessment for diagnostic purposes. Occasions might arise when the question is posed, "How is an individual's behavior affecting the good of the team?" Other issues I have encountered include coaching staff issues that are affecting team performance. In my work with USA Track and Field, the National Team staff is assigned based upon merit and service within the organization. Some have athletes on the team and some do not. All are usually head coaches at their respective institutions, and all are used to being the boss. One of the most valuable services that can be provided to this group of dedicated coaches is to help them become a team within a team. The pressures of the Olympic Games upon these individuals are immense. Some see this assignment as the capstone of their careers. All are dedicated to doing a great job and to helping the team succeed on one of the most visible stages in sport. I have found, along with my colleagues, that if we are to be successful as a team, a considerable amount of time must be devoted to this endeavor. The process begins a full two years prior to the games and involves the typical forming, storming, norming, and performing states of group. A consultant must have sufficient training to be able to handle this group of coaches as a facilitator as well as a member of the group. Such questions will arise as who is the client, who invited me into this setting, how do I best serve them, what is (are) the issue(s), where did they come from, what is the ultimate goal — to have a strong team, to win games, to win people, and what price is the team willing to pay for the goals set? The consultant must also be able to make decisions quickly in pressure situations. Sport does not always provide the time necessary to thoroughly discuss all options, and one must act quickly and well, or disaster might occur. Part of the solution comes from having a philosophy of service delivery that is set prior to the work with the team. Is your philosophy service or self-service? Are you the one onstage or are you willing to be offstage? Do you have strong foundational beliefs in the worth of each group member? Can you deal with the seduction of success and the agony of failure? Until a consultant has tested these beliefs in the heat of the competition, I do not believe he or she can be truly effective. Likewise, during the Olympic games is not a time for one to train and experiment with foundational beliefs.

In summary, it is important to meet the competency issue by knowing what we do not know. We should strive to maintain high standards of competence although recognizing our limitations and setting boundaries upon our use of techniques and intervention methods. We should continually seek opportunity for continuing education and take all appropriate precautions to protect the welfare of those with whom we work, whether individual or team sport athletes. Practicing beyond one's expertise is a serious breach of ethical boundaries.

Principle B: Integrity

One should seek to promote integrity in science, teaching, and practice of one's profession. Sport psychology consultants should be honest and fair in describing qualifications, services, products, and fees, and one should refrain from making statements that are false, misleading, or deceptive. To the extent feasible, one should clarify to all parties the roles they are performing and the obligations adopted. Especially, potentially harmful dual relationships should be avoided (paraphrased from Meyers, 1995).

The player-coach-sport psychologist relationship can be a very fruitful one. The key to making this work is to clarify from the onset the various roles. That is, who is the client? Who is paying the consulting fee? How do these activities interact and mesh? In the field of clinical or counseling psychology, these roles are usually identified and very few questions arise. In the field of sport, however, these roles can sometimes conflict with one another. If one has been hired by a sports franchise, is one part of management or an independent contractor? How is information transferred within the organization? When establishing my relationships within team sports, I operate on the premise that the athlete is my client. This is true even if the athletes do not pay my consultation fees directly. If management does not like this arrangement, then a referral is made to a colleague. This is the only ethical way for me to be effective. I do not consider myself part of management; rather my relationship to them is as an independent contractor. However, in team sports a consultant cannot alienate himself from management. If he does, he will find himself fired. There is some art to "walking a razor's edge" that does not fit cleanly into the established ethical principles. For instance, if management's goals start to interfere with the athlete's goals, the sport psychologist has a decision to make that is crucial to the success of the relationship. I always go back to my rule that the athlete is the client. I can use him or her as a clearinghouse for information without breaking coaching confidentiality. I have found that if an athlete trusts me and believes that I can help, then cooperation is easily conferred upon the consultant. However, my caution remains. One should not cross the coach in the role as coach without examining the consequences. Once again, this is an art more than a science. One must operate in an ethical framework while realizing that the sporting orientation and obligations are different from those in many other settings. A clear mission in sport, for instance, is winning. How does one cope with this? Philosophically a consultant must make clear his or her way of viewing the world of sport before entering the arena. If a consultant does not fully understand the consequences of viewing the sports world as it exists, then conflicts can constantly arise.

With the emergence of our field has come a competitive marketplace. Within this marketplace there have emerged consultants who have misrepresented their qualifications and expertise. It is essential that we protect our domain of practice. If we allow another agency to do so, we might lose our autonomy to practice. I often tell my classes and my audiences at national training camps any time I get the chance that if they meet a sport psychology consultant who promises miracles, then they must run as fast as they can in the other direction. This is where the referral process is important in our field. It is also extremely important to represent our services well and educate the various consumers well. I do not promise them anything except that together we will help them perform nearer their potential.

We must always seek to be honest, fair, and respectful of all people with whom we work; to clarify our roles as well as define the obligations we accept; and, finally, to avoid improper and potentially harmful dual relationships and conflicts of interest.

Principle C: Professional and Scientific Responsibility

Sport psychology consultants are responsible for safeguarding the public from those in the profession who are deficient in ethical conduct. They uphold professional standards of conduct and accept appropriate responsibility for their behavior. We consult with, refer to, or cooperate with other professionals and institutions to the extent needed to serve the best interests of the recipients of their services. We must safeguard the public's trust in our profession. When appropriate, we consult with colleagues in order to prevent, avoid, or terminate unethical conduct. In essence this is a personal as well as professional obligation for our field to survive with credibility. Professional organizations such as the AAASP and the APA Division 47 have taken the leadership role in establishing this trust. Very simply, we must conduct ourselves in such a way that it brings credit to the field. We do not exploit relationships with athletes for personal gain thorough media or publicity. We do not exploit relationships for personal gratification or jeopardize the safety and well-being of our clients, nor do we discriminate in any way.

It is my intent to put myself out of a job with a client. That is, a goal of mine is to make the client self-sufficient and independent. Once these athletes have achieved independence, then the relationship is appropriately terminated or altered. Coaches with whom I am consulting are the real sport psychologists. I am a consultant. Therefore, it seems logical that the role of mental consultant be turned over to the coaches and the athletes. I am truly a resource and therefore try very diligently not to establish a dependency model in the relationship. We do not terminate service prematurely; rather, we wean the coach and athlete to perform independently. I often joke that my eligibility has expired anyway. In my 25 years of consulting, one of the biggest errors I see in consultants is trying too hard to do too much. This is not done in a premeditated fashion but out of the need to help. I believe many of us fall several sigmas above the mean on the nurturance scale. It seems plausible that this could happen. This is where a well-placed consult with a colleague can contain the problem rather than leave it to fester and explode.

Principle D: Respect for People's Rights and Dignity

One of the greatest challenges is to mold a collection of individuals into a group without sacrificing all individuality to the group. One of the tasks faced by all coaches of team sports and sport psychologists working with team sports is to accomplish group synergy without sacrificing individual rights. One must be concerned with team goals and dreams as well as individual accomplishments and individual success within group success. I believe this is important in youth team sports as well as professional team sports. In youth sports, these emerging athletes are primarily involved to have fun. Yet, leaders are also concerned with group progress toward team goals. How does one balance the two ideals? In professional team sports, winning is the franchise goal. What are the goals of the members of the group? All of these concerns fall under respect for people's dignity and rights. In the field of sport there is a saying, "There is no I in team." However, we must remember there is an "I" in "Win." We must nourish the individual as well as the team.

Principle E: Concern for Other's Welfare

This principle requires the coach or sports consultant to have adequate training in group dynamics. Group facilitation, conflict-resolution skills, and communication facilitation are paramount to success in holding this principle in one's work. I do not know a single successful consultant or coach who is skilled and who completely abrogates his or her responsibilities in this area.

The sport psychologist is not coaching this athlete for a season or a career but for a lifetime. Once again, preparation and philosophical belief are the keys to successful consulting and coaching in this area.

Principle F: Social Responsibility

Sport psychology consultants accord appropriate respect to the fundamental rights, dignity, and worth of all people. They respect the rights to individual privacy, confidentiality, self-determination, and autonomy. Consultants also are aware of cultural, individual, and role differences with respect to age, ethnicity, race, gender, national origin, religion, sexual orientation, disability, language, and socioeconomic status. Consultants do not condone discrimination in any form. Also, consultants seek to contribute to the welfare of those with whom they interact in situations of power relationships in a professional way, and they are accountable to the community in which they work. Once again, these principles lead to being aware of exploitative relationships and complying with the law. Many ethical principles seem self-evident. However, unless one is cognizant and observant of one's behavior, then ethics can be overlooked. My credo over the years has been athletes first, winning second. Each of us needs to have these credos to live by. Sport ethics is an interesting area of study; Vernacchia (1990) has alluded to false sport ethics in his writings, and several of these are worth noting. The "I agree with you in principle, but..." sport ethic is of special note. As in any counseling relationship, what follows the "but" is usually the most interesting part of the statement. "The loophole ethic" is evident in the world of sport where to some the end justifies the means. The use of ergogenic aids supports the "high-tech/low conscience" ethic. All of us in the profession must operationalize our ethics and explore our own biases. If we do, we stand a very good chance of "being ethical."

Practical Suggestions

This chapter will conclude with practical suggestions for selecting a sport psychology consultant. These suggestions were developed by the AAASP (Association for the Advancement of Applied Sport Psychology, 1998). Athletes in team sports, as well as coaches of team sports, often are interested in contacting someone to help them with ethical decisions within the team sport context. Issues such as dealing with problematic athletes within team sport organizations, enhancing the moral and ethical orientation of youth sport athletes, and helping athletes make decisions related to life challenges are only a few reasons for contacting a sport psychology consultant regarding team sport issues. Consultants can provide information regarding communication issues, team building, cohesion factors, and motivation factors within groups, among other services. One of the best ways to select a qualified consultant is by word of mouth. Talking to athletes and coaches who have worked with a sport psychology professional provides an opportunity to hear about the qualifications of the ones who are good. Sport psychology professionals are somewhat like coaches in this regard. If they are asked back, then this is an excellent indicator of their effectiveness. Another way to obtain information is to consult a local university or athletic department, or to contact the major sport psychology organizations in one's country. In North America three excellent sources are the AAASP, APA Division 47, and the United States Olympic Committee Sport Psychology Registry.

In conclusion, each individual is responsible for his or her ethical behavior. We in the field of sport psychology are held to a high standard. This chapter has been an attempt to highlight these principles and to provide food for thought concerning this topic. The opportunity for growth is tremendous.

References

Association for the Advancement of Applied Sport Psychology. (1998). *Sport psychology: A guide to choosing a sport psychology professional.* Washington, DC: Author.

American Psychological Association. (1992). Ethical principles of psychologists and code of conduct. *The American Psychologist, 47,* 1597-1611.

Etzel, E., & Whelan, J. (1995). Considering ethics. *Association for the Advancement of Applied Sport Psychology, 10,* 25-26.

Henschen, K. (1997). Point-counterpoint: Using psychological assessment tools. *Association for the Advancement of Applied Sport Psychology, 12,* 15-16.

Meyers, A. (1995). Ethical principles of AAASP. *Association for the Advancement of Applied Sport Psychology, 10,* 15.

Nideffer, R. M. (1981). *The ethics and practice of applied sport psychology.* Ithaca, NY: Mouvement.

Petitpas, A. J., Brewer, B., Rivera, P., & Van Raalte, J. (1994). Ethical beliefs and behaviors in applied sport psychology: The AAASP ethics survey. *Journal of Applied Sport Psychology, 6,* 135-151.

Vernacchia, R. A. (1990, April). *The death of sport: Ethical concerns of drugs and performance.* A paper presented at the American Alliance for Health, Physical Education, Recreation and Dance National Convention, New Orleans, LA.

CHAPTER 4

Preperformance Routines in Self-Paced Tasks: Developmental and Educational Considerations

Ronnie Lidor and Robert N. Singer

Abstract

Empirical and anecdotal evidence suggests that preperformance routines are effective means for promoting physical and mental readiness prior to the execution of self-paced sport events. Whether such events occur in individual or team sports, the routines need to be performed systematically and consistently in order to facilitate learning and enhance performance. They help to create an ideal mental/psychological state prior to and during execution. Not surprisingly, good preperformance routines that are self-regulatory in nature are associated with skilled performance. However, to benefit from a particular routine, an individual should ideally experience and master it during the initial process of acquiring skill in any self-paced event. The purpose of this chapter is to examine developmental and educational considerations related to attaining proficiency in preperformance routines in young athletes who are involved in ball-game activities. These considerations reflect the psychological foundations needed to master self-paced skills as performed in real-game situations. Coaches should help athletes and athletes should help themselves in acquiring strategies and techniques that might contribute to a desirable preparatory routine.

> So I mentally tried to put myself in a familiar place. I thought about all those times I shot free throws in practice and went through the same motion, the same technique that I have used thousands of times. (Jordan, 1994, p. 11)
>
> . . . But whatever your preparation, establish a routine . . . whatever your routine is, go through it before each free throw.
> (Bird, 1986, p. 50)

Virtually all skilled athletes who are involved in sports that contain brief self-paced events have preperformance routines, either taught or intuitively developed. Self-paced acts are those taking place in a relatively stable and predictable environment, where there is adequate time to prepare for the execution (Singer, 1988, 2001). In these, the person can activate a plan, a strategy, a protocol, a procedure, a preshot routine, a ritual, or what we are terming a preperformance routine. The goal is to facilitate learning, performance, and achievement. Effective preperformance routines are usually mastered with a high degree of consistency. That is, either deliberately or subconsciously (depending on level of skill), they become an integral part of the sport act itself.

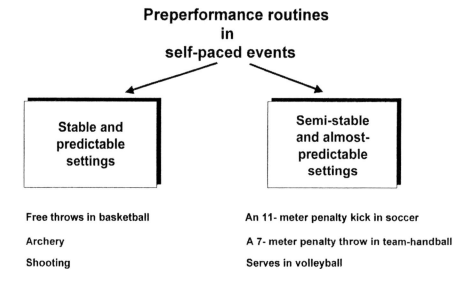

Figure 1. Preperformance routines as part of stable and semistable settings

Examples of self-paced events are diving, weight lifting, bowling, golf, and archery. Other examples are the free throw in basketball and the serve in tennis. In these events, the settings are stable, predictable, and anticipated, and the individual can carry out a specific plan. However, preperformance routines can also be used in semistable and almost-predictable settings, as illustrated in Figure 1. For example, in performing the 11-meter penalty kick in soccer and the 7-meter penalty throw in team handball, the athlete who stands on the line has to consider the stance of the goalkeeper and potential movements before the act takes place. Although one of the conditions in these events is not stable and not easy to anticipate (the goalkeeper's actions), the attacker can plan an act and activate it as it had originally been structured. In both stable and semistable environments, the athlete can use a routine in which control over motor, emotional, and cognitive behaviors is attained. For the purpose of this chapter, both stable and semistable self-paced acts are considered for implementing relevant preperformance routines.

Preperformance routines, depending on the person and the sport, may occur for a relatively brief period (e.g., 5-20 sec.) before the initiation of the act. By developing a personalized and meaningful routine, the athlete feels more in control over what he or she is about to do and, therefore, the performance outcome (Cohn, 1990). The routine encompasses movements, thoughts, and emotions prior to "action," or even during the action, with the intention of optimizing the preparatory state and execution capabilities of the athlete.

Various aspects of such routines, as well as total routines, have been studied as to how they contribute to achievement. They are well documented in the sport psychology literature (e.g., Cohn, 1990; Singer, Hausenblas, & Jannelle, 2001; Singer, Murphey, & Tennant, 1993; Southard, Miracle, & Landwer, 1989; Wrisberg & Pain, 1992) and sometimes with anecdotes (Bird, 1986; Jordan, 1994; Louganis, 1995). Consistent and effective routines are associated with acquiring motor skills more efficiently, as well as with demonstrating the highest level of expertise. Those who follow great divers remember Greg Louganis' magnificent dives at two Olympics (1984 and 1988) and his ability to be completely focused before each dive. Karl Malone, the perennial All-Star American professional basketball player and winner of the most valuable player award in the 1998-99 season, exhibits a unique systematic ritual before shooting a free throw. Ronaldo, the fantastic Brazilian soccer player, has refined his preparatory technique over years of practice for use in a situation that requires the 11-meter penalty kick.

The general purpose of a performance routine is to put oneself in an optimally aroused, self-expectant, confident, and focused state immediately prior to, as well as during, execution. In a sense, self-regulatory techniques are essential (Carver & Scheier, 1998; Crews, 1993; Hardy & Nelson, 1988). They are used to control and direct emotions, thoughts, and attention so that ideal inner harmony is present. For golfers, it is having the feeling and timing that enables great shots to be made. The athlete is then more likely to produce the act at a performance level compatible with his or her true capabilities. Many athletes, especially those under severe competitive stress, may handicap themselves with self-doubt and too much tension and distraction, as well as fear of failing, looking bad, or letting down significant others. The preperformance routine is an enabler. That is to say, it should enable an individual to trust him/herself and to become immersed in the performance situation with the belief and feeling that the execution will go well.

However, to effectively use preperformance routines in sport, one should acquire these techniques as early as possible during the process of learning the sport itself. If the techniques of the skills are acquired at an early age (Christina & Corcos, 1988), then the preparation routines that are performed in combination with these techniques should be taught to the learner in early stages of the training as well. Unfortunately, both the scientific and applied literature do not provide any suggestions, recommendations, and implications on how to (a) teach preperformance routines to young learners, (b) incorporate these routines with the execution of the act, and (c) integrate the routines under competitive sport situations.

The following two observations may provide more insight into these shortcomings in the literature. These instructional cases are taken from team sport activities. However, both are considered as self-paced events.

Case 1. Michael is a 17-year-old basketball player on a high school team. He arrives at the gym about 45 minutes before the practice begins. He wants to spend more time on his free-throw shots. In the last game he did poorly when standing on the line; he made the basket only 4 times of 10 attempts. He knows that 40% success from the foul line will not give him too many opportunities to play for the team.

When he practices free-throw shots, he tries to develop a preperformance routine. He has been told by his coach to "do the same thing before each of the shots." However, he fails to do this. In his first attempt, he bounces the ball twice in the readying state before shooting, and in the following attempt he bounces it four times. In one attempt he focuses his eyes at the front area of the rim, but during the next few attempts his concentration wanders. He feels that he is losing his focus. He starts missing the shot time after time. Michael cannot organize his thoughts "in the right direction." He feels anxious, and he is looking for his coach's assistance. However, Phil (the coach) has not yet arrived. Michael gives up. He is sitting on the bench waiting for practice to officially begin.

Case 2. Laurie is a 14-year-old soccer player. She is a member of the school's team. She works hard during practices and tries her best not to miss any. Because of her high motivation during workouts and games, she was nominated as the captain of the team. One of her responsibilities is to perform the 11-meter penalty kick. She likes to do it because she likes to score. She enjoys the "competitive edge" between herself and the goalkeeper: Only the two of them are in the center of the scene. She knows that if she scores, she will be the hero of the game.

Although Laurie is doing fairly well in her kicking performances, she does not feel comfortable during the period of time she needs to prepare herself for the penalty kick. It seems to her that she changes her routine before every kick. One time she runs very fast and, without any hesitation, kicks the ball. In another attempt, she runs at a slow pace without knowing exactly at what side of the goal she is going to aim. She feels that she has little control over what she is doing and therefore lacks confidence in producing effective kicks. Laurie asks her coach for advice. She is told to "just relax and concentrate on what you are doing." She tries to apply this suggestion. However, she feels that not much guidance has been given to her. She continues to feel uncertain about how she should prepare herself during penalty-kick situations.

The purpose of this chapter is to examine the effectiveness of preperformance routines in self-paced acts performed by young athletes such as Michael and Laurie who are involved in team sport activities such as ball games. More specifically, developmental and educational considerations are elaborated upon in order to assist coaches and instructors in guiding young athletes how to implement preperformance routines. The appropriate use of learning and performance strategies is emphasized.

There are six parts in this chapter. First, a brief overview of the literature is provided on the use of preperformance routines in sport. In the second part, a learning strategy is defined, followed by a description of two practical strategies that can be used by the learners in their attempts to develop preperformance routines. The psychological and psychophysiological factors contributing to success in self-spaced skills are discussed in the third and fourth part, respectively. In the fifth part, developmental and educational considerations are suggested for the coach and the athlete to assist them in effectively structuring preperformance routines. Among these considerations are (a) using kinesthetic feedback in controlling emotions and behaviors, (b) focusing attention, and (c) providing self-feedback information. Examples of these considerations are offered with respect to the two instructional cases mentioned earlier in this chapter. Finally, in the sixth part, seven practical recommendations are provided for the coach and the instructor.

Preperformance Routines in Self-Paced Tasks: A Brief Overview of the Literature

A preperformance routine has been defined as a systematic sequence of motor, emotional, and cognitive behaviors that are demonstrated on a regular basis immediately before the execution of self-paced tasks (Gould & Udry, 1994; Moran, 1996). The routine is part of an athlete's repertoire when preparing to perform. Athletes and coaches generally believe that the to-be-performed act should be enhanced by the ability to generate a routine that provides the athlete with an optimal functioning state.

According to some scholars (e.g., Cohn, 1990; Moran, 1996; Southard & Miracle, 1993), the initiation of relevant preperformance routines should be beneficial, particularly in attempts to "stay focused" and to be "under control" before and during movement execution. Although each athlete demonstrates a personalized systematic sequence of motor behaviors, such as the stance and how the ball is bounced before the penalty throw in team handball or the serve in volleyball, the goal is to develop a psychological edge in performance. Much more goes on in the routine besides the observable physical behaviors, namely in the head!

Among the benefits of a well-developed preperformance routine in sport are (a) enhancing the process of focusing attention, (b) preventing negative thoughts and reflections, (c) blocking external distractions, and (d) developing a plan of action before the performance begins (Moran, 1996). Above all, this preparation ritual provides the performer with the feeling that he or she is in optimal control of what is going on, thereby facilitating achievement. Singer and Chen (1994) and Chen and Singer (1992) have offered suggestions for the use of cognitive strategies in contributing to self-regulation and perception of control prior to and during performance.

Research on the usefulness of preparation routines in sport has indicated that learners who were taught how to implement systematic routines associated with the performance of self-paced activities such as the free throw in basketball achieved better and more consistently compared with those who were not exposed to these guidelines (Lobmeyer & Wasserman, 1986; Wrisberg & Anshel, 1989). Among the routines that were administered to participants in such studies were mental imagery and arousal adjustment (Wrisberg & Anshel, 1989), relaxation (Lamirand & Rainey, 1994), and visual-motor behavior rehearsal (VMBR; Hall & Erffmeyer, 1983). In general, those who were taught how to use one of these mental techniques were able to attain a higher level of proficiency in comparison with those who were not trained how to use them.

Not surprisingly, preperformance routines were taught only after the participants in the investigations had some experience with the pertinent sport skills. One of the most popular skills studied is the free-throw shot in basketball (Lobmeyer & Wasserman, 1986; Wrisberg & Anshel, 1989). Before being guided how to use a preparatory technique such as imagery, participants had already acquired the fundamentals of the shot. The mental technique was taught to them at a point when they had probably played basketball on numerous occasions and had learned the shot to a reasonable degree. In this kind of a learning process, the learners are trying to make a match between a "newly acquired knowledge," for instance, a preparation routine, and "an already-acquired knowledge," for example, shooting a free throw in basketball.

The effectiveness of a preparatory routine presented to learners during their initial attempts in acquiring a new self-paced motor task has generally not been examined by researchers. The components of a preperformance routine should be introduced to learners as part of the instructional guidelines associated with technical information about how to execute the skill. The combined set of instructions, the techniques for performing the sport skill, and the preparatory technique should be offered at the very beginning phase of the learning process.

It is true that in some studies (e.g., Southard & Miracle, 1993; Wrisberg & Pain, 1992), researchers have observed the preperformance rituals of skilled performers in order to study systematic patterns of behaviors demonstrated by those who are tops in their area of expertise. However, those routines used by skilled athletes may not be appropriate for beginning learners. The beginner obviously lacks experience and skill and thus needs to acquire semantic and procedural knowledge compatible with existing knowledge and capabilities. In other words, knowing what to do and how to do it under different conditions reflects the refinement of performance techniques and self-regulatory strategies (Lidor, 1999; Singer, 2001).

Cohn (1990), in an extensive review of the literature on theoretical and practical applications of preperformance routines in sport, has provided sport-specific guidelines for helping beginners to develop such routines. However, it seems that not much attention has been given to the implementation of preperformance routines in the early stages of learning sport skills. A learner should benefit considerably by mastering a meaningful preparatory strategy as early as possible during the learning experience.

In addition, Wrisberg and Pain (1992) have argued that "the athlete should be allowed the freedom to develop a ritual that is subjectively most comfortable" (p. 22). Whether a beginner or a serious performer, personal factors must be considered as to the comfort and effectiveness in performance production. This suggestion is most important at early stages of learning, when preperformance routines may be more easily modified, adapted, and developed. When refined, task learning and performance benefits should be efficiently demonstrated and long-lasting. The point that is emphasized in this chapter is that preperformance routines can and should be experienced, learned, and used during every stage of developing skill in a self-paced sport activity. Appropriate instructional strategies are necessary. Among the strategies that should assist learners in developing the mechanics of the movements constituting the sport or act in a sport are those that help ready an athlete to be in an optimal emotional/mental state to execute. We suggest that a preperformance routine can be taught simultaneously with the mechanics of the sport skills, without allocating a great deal of additional time and effort.

A Learning Strategy Approach

A type of instructional technique that is useful for developing preperformance routines at the very initial phase of the learning process is a learning strategy. A learning strategy has been defined as a form of guidance for learners in acquiring skills, as well as an approach that should be helpful in selecting performance strategies and building or repairing them (Lidor, 1999; Singer, 1988, 2001). A. Anderson (1997) has postulated that learning strategies are the cognitive tools used to systematically manage the thought processes associated with knowledge and skill acquisition. Such strategies are usually externally directed by a coach or teacher or, more ideally, self-initiated in appropriate situations (Singer, 1978; Singer & Gershon, 1979).

Considering these perspectives, a broad learning strategy is the overall plan one formulates for accomplishing personal achievement goals and the knowledge about the usefulness of this plan for this purpose. In addition, more specific strategies are related to the behaviors and thoughts that a learner activates either deliberately or subconsciously during learning in an attempt to influence information-processing processes, and in turn the level of achievement in an activity.

Research in educational psychology has indicated that achievement in academic tasks such as reading comprehension, writing, memorizing a series of events, and solving problems is positively influenced by using relevant strategies (e.g., Weinstein & Mayer, 1986). Educational psychologists such as Gardner (1983), Sternberg (1985), and Perkins (1992) believe that broad strategies can enhance the ability of students to acquire self-management and self-evaluation skills, which in turn will affect their ability to develop independence throughout the learning process. Similar observations can also be found in the psychomotor domain.

The effectiveness of learning strategies has been examined in the learning and performance of closed (self-paced) movement skills. In a series of laboratory (e.g., Lidor, Tennant, & Singer, 1996; Singer, Lidor, & Cauraugh, 1993, 1994) and field (e.g., Lidor, 1997; Lidor, Arnon, & Bronstein, 1999) studies, task-pertinent learning strategies have been shown to enhance accuracy in dart throwing, ball throwing, bowling, and free-throw shots. Participants in these studies were shown how to implement the principles of the strategies, prior to having any meaningful experience with the to-be-learned task. More important, they were exposed to pre- and during-performance strategy guidance at the time that they were explained how to execute the task. They were provided with technical and strategy instructions before being asked to perform. Practically speaking, they used the strategy information as a preperformance routine.

Among the many and varied strategies that have been reported and advocated in the literature (e.g., Singer et al., 1993, 1994) are the five-step approach (5-SA) and the awareness strategy (AS) for learning and performing self-paced motor skills. These instructional strategies have the potential to assist learners in developing meaningful pre- and during-performance routines at the very initial phase of the learning process. In addition, they are easy to use as an integral part of any technical information offered about the execution of a sport act.

For the purpose of this chapter, only the 5-SA is elaborated upon and discussed in detail, and its applicability in structuring preperformance routines by beginning learners is demonstrated. The AS is briefly presented because of its instructional potential to assist beginners in increasing their awareness of performance upon acquiring the mechanics of the skill. It is recommended that the coach apply the AS only when the instructional time is limited. Although the 5-SA is a more comprehensive, time-consuming, and complicated technique than the AS, our recommendation is to implement the 5-SA as the main approach while developing preperformance routines related to stable and semistable self-paced events.

The Five-Step Approach

The 5-SA is a global learning and performance strategy that is composed of the following sequential steps: readying, imaging, focusing attention, executing, and evaluating (Singer, 1988). This strategy is relatively content independent and designed to improve learning and performance in all motor tasks classified as self-paced. The components of the strategy are presented in Figure 2.

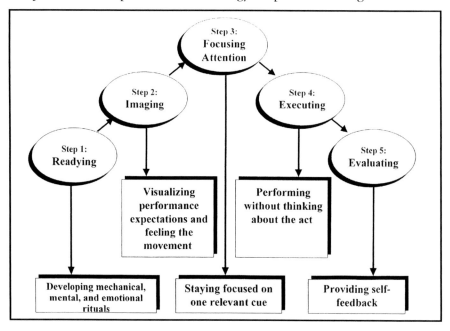

Figure 2. The five-step approach as an educational technique for the development of preperformance routines

During the readying step, learners are taught how to be mentally, emotionally, mechanically, and physically prepared to execute at their best. For example, they need to know how to monitor, as well as to control and direct, emotions and motivations for realizing an optimal arousal condition for the task to be learned in a neutral setting and performed in a competitive setting. In the imaging step, learners are directed how to visualize themselves performing the act and its outcome to the best of their ability. They are guided how to feel the rhythm of the movement while they mentally picture themselves completing the act according to their capabilities at that time in their development.

During the focusing-attention step, the importance of narrowing concentration to one relevant thought or cue in the performance setting, such as the target center in archery or shooting, is emphasized. By applying this process, internal or external distractors should be blocked. In the executing step, the idea is to perform without thinking of the act or the outcome of the act. Learners are told to "just do it," as if in a state of automaticity. They have to learn to trust themselves in order to be able to execute without thinking about the execution. In the evaluating step, learners are guided to use their own movement-generated feedback as well as results to evaluate their performance, if time is available. Evaluation not only has to do with the outcome of the act, but also whether each of the steps in the 5-SA was implemented appropriately. These stages will be elaborated on shortly.

The transition in attention was explained in the classic work of Schnieder and Shiffrin (1977), in which automated and controlled processes were differentiated. Automatic processes, as compared with controlled processes, are rapid, effortless, and consistent, among other characteristics (Logan, 1988). In very difficult tasks or those that are not well learned, controlled processes (nonautomatic) are usually required. Attention is allocated to various aspects of the situation and performance.

The first three steps of the strategy—readying, imaging, and focusing attention—are preparatory to initiating the movement act. The next step deals with quieting the mind during execution. The final step occurs when the act is completed. Therefore, in reality, the 5-SA encompasses preparatory, during, and post-act considerations, all of which are important for achievement. With practice, these stages can be completed with apparent automaticity.

The Awareness Strategy

The AS is an approach associated with paying attention to kinesthetic cues, feeling of the movements, and thinking about the act while performing (Clark & Norch, 1986; Lidor, 1999; Singer et al., 1994). This strategy directs learners to be aware of body sensations while the movement is being carried out. They are told that they will be provided with appropriate directions on how to pay attention to body parts and sensations as the act is performed. Kinesthetic information is explained so that they can feel their movements and use self-feedback information for improving their next attempts in executing the act.

According to this strategy, learners should plan an awareness routine before the act and then activate it during the movement. The AS is supposed to assist them to develop awareness of what to do before performance as well as during performance. To implement this strategy, learners are instructed to

1. Feel their movements.
2. Think about the act.
3. Pay attention to small details.
4. Be aware of what they are doing.

Focusing on body awareness of the task while it is being performed is thought to be one of the soundest procedures in learning a sport routine. Presumably, the more the person is aware of what is happening during the performance, the more he or she is able to develop a correct routine associated with skilled performance. Individuals may increase their awareness of the correct way to execute a skill. However, it should be pointed out that the AS is a learning strategy for beginners. Experts, who perform with automaticity, presumably do not pay attention to the process of the act. They "just do it," when everything is going well.

Both the 5-SA and the AS for the learning of self-paced motor skills are thought to provide appropriate tools to structure preperformance and during-performance routines related to the execution of self-paced sport acts. There are similarities and differences between the 5-SA and the AS. Particularly, the 5-SA is a more global strategy that can be implemented not only before but also after performance. More important, the first three preparatory steps of the 5-SA--readying, imaging, and focusing attention--include awareness components related to the act and the environment. In fact, it has been argued by Lidor (1999) that the 5-SA contains both awareness and nonawareness (i.e., the fourth step of the strategy) components of behavioral and cognitive routines. Considering this comparison as well as empirical evidence favoring the use of the 5-SA (e.g., Lidor et al., 1996; Singer et al., 1993, 1994), we consider the 5-SA to be more useful in learning and performing self-paced acts.

The main reason for this is that the strategy contains elements thought to be important in achieving self-paced sport skills demonstrated in game situations. If such a learning strategy as the 5-SA can benefit the learner during beginning stages in the learning process, then it should also be of benefit to routines executed in real-game situations. When the psychological demands of self-paced skills on those competing in a game situation are considered, the 5-SA should contribute to performance effectiveness.

Psychological Factors Contributing to Success

When examining the psychological demands on an athlete preparing for the performance of a self-paced activity, such as a weight lifter, diver, or shooter, or those in game situations, such as John Stockton readying himself for the free-throw shot, Zinadin Zidan planning a penalty kick in soccer, or Pete Sampras organizing his thoughts and emotions before unleashing a wicked serve, the three main characteristics most likely to appear are

1. Readying oneself consistently as to mechanical, mental, and emotional considerations,
2. Focusing attention appropriately immediately prior to and during the act, and
3. Evaluating (if time permits).

These behaviors are part of any performance routine activated in particular game situations by a basketball player, a tennis player, a soccer player, and others. We will now elaborate on them.

Readying. The person must be mechanically, mentally, and psychologically prepared to perform at his or her best. A systematic sequence of behaviors contributes to the successful demonstration of the act. These must be practiced repeatedly over a period of time, so as to become automatic. The overall routine should help to contribute to feelings of control over general expectations as well as the execution and outcome of the act.

It seems that such "hidden behaviors," or mental and psychological readiness, are very challenging to master and difficult to control, especially under stressful situations. However, they are necessary in order to realize optimal arousal, concentration, and confidence states (Weinberg & Gould, 1999). In addition, the movements associated with the act, the movement plan, should be constructed prior to action. It is desirable to convince oneself of one's ability to successfully execute the task, to trust oneself. It is well known (Bandura, 1997) that self-efficacy influences how people feel, think, act, and accomplish in specific activities. Thus, actual performance is related to one's belief in personal competence.

Focusing Attention. In self-paced tasks, performance occurs in a stable and predictable setting. Attention should be narrowed and directed to a target (e.g., the front area of the rim in shooting a free throw) or a zone (e.g., the opponent's zone of serving in volleyball). Apparently, the ability to be focused prior to and during an action is crucial in determining proficiency. Athletes have time to select the appropriate cue and to appropriately focus attention. When the same activity is repeated under similar conditions, they should be able to develop an optimal state of concentration. This process by itself should lead to a reduced negative effect of any potential internal distractors (self-doubt) or external distractors (noise, movement of others), thereby resulting in better performance. Our research indicates the preferability of directing attention to an external cue (like the target) rather than to one's movements, as described earlier in the self-awareness strategy (Singer et al., 1993, 1994).

The act of focusing attention on a cue should assist the performer to (a) reduce information-processing activity, (b) block out any potential distractors (internal or external), and (c) perform the task without conscious attention, as if in a state of automaticity, as experts apparently do. Some common distractions to performance are feelings of self-doubt, fear of failure, and fear of performing badly, as well as being too aware of the pressure of others, noise, and other distracting factors.

Evaluating. Although the evaluation process is not part of the preperformance routine in sport, it is an essential aspect of achievement. The use of knowledge of performance outcomes, as well as an analysis of contributors to the performance outcome, is necessary for improvement in skill. If time permits, a person should analyze the outcome of his or her performance and the process leading to it, in-between attempts at execution. In self-paced ball-sport events, performers are aware of the outcome of their performance. Experienced athletes understand, when unsuccessful, what they need to do differently and better in future attempts. For example, when good tennis players serve unsuccessfully, they are able to (a) analyze the potential causes for the outcome and (b) reflect on a better way to serve next time, taking into consideration mechanical and psychological factors. Self-feedback can be used without any dependence on an external source, such as a coach or instructor, if the individual knows how to analyze effectively. That knowledge will be useful in future attempts.

The psychological foundations for achieving, readiness, focusing attention, and evaluating should be introduced when young people are attempting to acquire a skill. They should be provided with specific guidelines on what they have to do in order to cope with and overcome potential mental and psychological barriers that may arise immediately before and during execution. Developmental and educational considerations for structuring preperformance routines are discussed later. In addition, specific considerations to assist Michael (Case 1) and Laurie (Case 2) to overcome their performance obstacles will be suggested. These educational guidelines are based upon the introduction of a learning strategy (such as the 5-SA) combined with the technical information provided to the learner at the initial phase of the learning.

Psychophysiological Contributors to Success

In another direction, self-paced skills such as rifle shooting, archery, and golf have been the subject of psychophysiological research to determine profiles of experts when they execute, as well as when they perform at their best. Strategy implications have been derived from this type of research as to how to perform better by being in an ideal state immediately prior to and during the act. Other areas of interest have been electrical activity in the brain, respiration rate, heart rate (HR), EMG activity, and visual search patterns.

Electroencephalogram (EEG) wave patterns, especially with regard to alpha level immediately prior to and during execution, presumably represent an important index reflecting attentional processing. Each hemisphere is associated with different processing activities such as the left for analytical-verbal and the right for spatial. Conflicting research findings (Hatfield, Landers, & Ray, 1987; Landers et al., 1994) associated with highly skilled athletes have been reported in regard to alpha activity in either or both hemispheres. More alpha activity in the left hemisphere, to a point, might be related to less active verbal-analytical processes. Thus, the athlete's state would ideally be to "let it happen" in order to produce an act without deliberate awareness. For instance, Hatfield, Landers, and Ray (1984) studied elite marksmen and found an increase in alpha activity in the left hemisphere within 7.5 sec. of pulling the trigger. Alpha activity in the right hemisphere remained constant. In another study, Salazar et al. (1990) analyzed the four best and worst shots of archers and noted that an increase in alpha activity in the left hemisphere was related to poorer performances. Perhaps too little or too much alpha activity contributes to undermining achievement potential.

Lacey (1967) has proposed that HR decelerates and cortical activity lessens immediately before one initiates an act that requires an external attentional focus, such as in target-aiming tasks. Putting in golf, archery, and rifle shooting have been used to test Lacey's hypothesis. To provide further perspectives with regard to alpha activity, HR, and performance, Radlo et al. (2002) also examined the effects of an internal focusing strategy versus an external one on dart-throwing skill. The external group (focusing on the center of the target) performed better than the other group, which was taught to direct attention toward self-movements when making a toss. HR decelerated in the external group immediately prior to dart release, although the opposite was true for the other group. EEG alpha power was lower for the external group. Implications are that an external strategy leads to more ideal psychophysiological functions that enable better skilled performance.

Radlo (1997) also compared the effects of the 5-SA on developing skill in a dart-throwing task under noncompetitive and competitive conditions. EEG activity and HR were assessed immediately before and during tosses. This strategy not only led to significantly better performance scores than those in the control group, but also to increased alpha activity and decreased beta activity in the left hemisphere. The opposite occurred with the control group. This strategy apparently led to the right side of the brain's becoming the dominant processor, thereby minimizing distracting verbal/analytical information. In addition to a decrease in left hemisphere activation, the strategy led to progressive HR deceleration in the 5-SA group, whereas the control group showed increased HR immediately prior to the release of the dart. The emphasis on the strategy to focus attention externally on the target seemed to be related to the decelerated HR and was consistent with other research (Boutcher & Zinsser, 1990; Lacey, 1967). In addition to comparisons made between the strategy group and the control group, the four best and worst shots were analyzed according to the Mean Radial Error (MRE) scores. Best achievement was associated with an increase in alpha activity in the left hemisphere and a decrease in HR immediately before the toss.

Visual search, or gaze, behaviors have been assessed in other research to determine differences between experts and novices in such activities as billiards, putting in golf, and free-throw shooting in basketball. Fixation duration and location data imply the degree of focus of attention (concentration) immediately prior to and during the act. For target skills, the extent of concentration on the critical point of aim is of interest. In billiards and putting in golf, gaze patterns shift back and forth until the player is ready to actually perform the skill. Another consideration is the quantity of time spent in the preparation phase to execute, depending on task complexity, and comparing times of experts with those less skilled. This theme will be discussed shortly. These kinds of evidence imply strategies that performers may want to use to improve their preparatory/attentional skills. Consistency is a great contributor to level of performance as well.

Duration of fixation on a target preparatory to the movement act has been termed "quiet eye" duration by Vickers (1996). Presumably, longer quiet-eye periods lead to better performance, and parameters, or movement requirements, are set during this time. This internal activity, also termed cognitive processing (response programming), would be longer for more complex tasks (e.g., Henry & Rogers, 1960). In essence, visual control over movement skill in target-aiming tasks seems to be a critical consideration (Vickers, 1996).

As to the quiet eye duration, Vickers (1996, 1997) tested the Canadian women's national basketball team and found that the more highly skilled free-throw shooters differed from the less skilled. Better shooters were recorded with durations of almost 900 ms whereas the less-skilled average less than 400 ms. Frehlich (1997) observed similar data with billiard players. Three shots standardized as to degree of increasing difficulty yielded data of 500 ms versus 275 ms comparing two groups of players with different levels of skill. Vickers (1996) also noted that the expert shooters spent more time in preparing for the shot. However, in a study conducted by Frehlich (1997), the two groups of billiard players did not differ in time allotment.

Also analyzed in putting in golf (Vickers, 1992) and in billiards play (Frehlich, 1997) were fixation patterns to different locations. In both studies, experts seemed to fixate on only a few important locations. Shifting in gaze patterns in billiards, that is, on the cue ball, to the object ball, and back to the cue ball, was similar between the groups. However, the novice group repeated the sequence more frequently, and spent less time at each location as well. The more highly skilled players are characterized as having more efficient scan paths, as suggested by Abernethy (1988), than those of skilled performers in general.

In summary, it is becoming more obvious that the study of the behavioral and psychophysiological aspects of expertise, as well as experimental manipulations in the adoption of particular useful strategies, provide important information for understanding how to perform self-paced tasks more capably. Refinement in the use of attentional and cognitive processes leads to more skilled performance.

Developmental and Educational Considerations: General and Specific

While working with young beginners, coaches or instructors should consider their learning and performance capabilities, as well as their expectations (Christina & Corcos, 1988; Singer, 1986). Motor skill research has provided useful information as to how to acquire and master motor skills (Schmidt & Lee, 1999; Schmidt & Wrisberg, 2000; Singer, 1980). Many guidelines are related to practice arrangements (Lee, Chamberlin, & Hodges, 2001) and the content of the activity (Christina & Corcos, 1988). However, to enhance strategic behavior of young people at an early stage of the learning process, coaches and instructors should be particularly knowledgeable about the beginners' information-processing and attentional capabilities.

It has been well established in the research literature that age, maturational level, and experience are important considerations in the ability of children to analyze task-performance situations, select appropriate cues, organize and generate plans for a movement, memorize a series of movements, and use ongoing feedback (Gallagher & Thomas, 1986; Nevett & French, 1997; Singer, 1986). But, research evidence has shown (McPherson, 1993) that children at various ages, such as a 12-year-old, can learn to improve upon information-processing capabilities and to make capacities more functional, within developmental limitations. In other words, young learners can develop more useful strategies if they are taught how to do so.

Therefore, coaches are encouraged to assist young beginners in structuring preperformance routines in two practical ways. First, coaches should introduce the components of the strategy as part of the technical guidelines of the skill, in order to create a vivid link between the technique and the strategy. Second, they should teach one cognitive component at a time, like focusing attention, in order to decrease the cognitive load imposed on the learners.

A global strategy for learning and performing self-paced motor tasks, such as the 5-SA, can promote "good" routines related to readiness (physical and mental), confidence building (imaging), attention focusing, and evaluating. As a result, achievement should be facilitated. The components of this or related strategies, if they are integrated with the technical information offered (for example, the basic foundations of a free throw in basketball) to the learner at the initial phase of the learning, should provide the best experiences.

Throughout the process of learning, the learner would ideally be introduced to the psychological foundations of achieving, one at a time, as illustrated in Figure 3. A young beginner does not have sufficient experience with the skill to be mastered. He or she will pay attention mainly to the technique of performing the skill, so it is probably more advantageous to develop only one aspect of the preparatory routine at a time. After some experience with attempting to accomplish the task, as well as with mastering a particular psychological contributor to success, the learner might be able to acquire another strategy, such as evaluating. Gradually, all components of the preperformance and during-performance routine are learned, along with the proper execution of the task itself.

Every coach should know that "good teaching" includes teaching students not only how to perform, but also how to learn, how to remember, how to think, and how to motivate themselves. Task-relevant strategies help to improve these capabilities. Furthermore, strategies such as the 5-SA can provide learners with the cognitive means not only to perform the act as it has been acquired in a sterile learning environment (as it is in typical practice environments), but also to adapt to a more challenging situation (as it exists in a competitive game).

In other words, good strategies can enhance the acquisition of declarative knowledge (what to do), and facilitate the implementation of procedural knowledge (when to do it and how to do it) (J. R. Anderson, 1990).

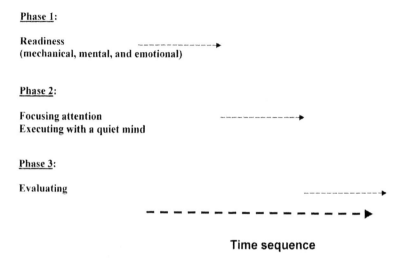

Figure 3. Developmental phases in structuring preperformance routines over time

From an educational perspective, providing learners with technical and strategic information may increase the cognitive load put on them at the initial phase of the learning process. They will be required to pay attention to small details related to the mechanics of the skill, such as how to release the ball in free-throw shots or how to make the football contact in the 11-meter kick in soccer, and at the same time to implement the principles of the strategy, such as how to focus attention at the front area of the rim or the abdominal zone of the goalkeeper. This combined instructional approach might initially slow down the learning process. However, it might enable learners to refine their ability to process information related to mastering the activity and adapting to game situations in the long run.

General guidance. Instructional and developmental considerations are presented for the three phases associated with an ideal routine: readying, focusing attention, and evaluating (See Table 1). In each phase, the steps of the 5-SA are outlined. The components of the strategy are introduced in relation to the psychological characteristics outlined earlier in this chapter, namely readiness, focusing attention, and evaluating. In order to match between the components of the strategy and the psychological contributors to success in self-paced tasks, the readying and imaging stages are combined. The combined stages should assist beginners to effectively develop the mechanical, mental, and emotional aspects of the readiness routine conducted a short period of time before execution.

Instruction for each psychological foundation should be integrated within the technical guidance given to the learner by the coach or instructor. However, such experiences should be specified according to the task, situation, and skill and age level of the performer.

Specific guidance. To demonstrate how guidance should be applied to a specific situation, guidelines for each psychological foundation are provided separately for Case 1 (free-throw performance; Table 2) and Case 2 (an 11-meter penalty kick; Table 3). In Case 1, Michael has the opportunity to repeatedly execute the task in a game situation, that is, shooting two times in a row, if he is fouled in the act of shooting. However, in Case 2, Laurie can perform only once due to the fact that immediately after the kicking attempt, the game is continued. The foundations of the readiness and focusing attention phases can be applied similarly in both cases. However, the immediate evaluating process can be activated only in Case 1.

It was observed in Case 1 that Michael had difficulties in his readiness approach to shooting the basketball. He should be taught how to develop a preparatory routine. He probably will benefit most from the guidelines suggested in the first phase of the preparatory ritual.

Phase	Psychological Foundation	Emphasis	Guidelines	5-SA
I	readying (mechanical, mental, and emotional)	directing thoughts and emotions to create an optimal state for learning and/or performing; imaging the act vividly	- establishing a consistent basic position - feeling comfortable in the position - generating positive thoughts and emotions about performance expectations - creating confidence - developing awareness of what needs to be done: An action plan - visualizing best possible personal performance - feeling the movements to be performed - developing awareness of body parts during execution	Steps 1 and 2: readying and imaging

Table 1. Instructional and developmental considerations for developing an ideal routine

Phase	Psychological Foundation	Emphasis	Guidelines	5-SA
II	focusing attention	selecting a relevant external cue and focusing intently on it	- focusing attention on one situational cue or thought - maintaining only this thought - blocking out internal thoughts, such as "I hope I won't miss the shot"; "I wish I weren't here"; "I hope I don't let down the team" - blocking out external distractors, such as: * the presence of others * "trash talk" of opponents * flashing cameras * weather conditions - executing with a quiet mind	Step 3: focusing attention
III	evaluating	using self-feedback for analysis and subsequent improvement	- judging the outcome of the performance - assessing the processes and strategies that produced the movement - determining better ways to perform in the future, if appropriate	Step 5: evaluating

* Note: Appropriate use of the strategy can also assist performers in developing a mechanical routine.

Table 1. Instructional and developmental considerations for developing an ideal routine

Phase	Psychological Foundation	Guidelines	5-SA
I	readying (mechanical, mental, and emotional)	- stepping up to the foul line; setting the feet, getting into a comfortable position - holding the ball; getting the feeling of the ball - bouncing the ball a couple of times (or more) - bringing the ball to the shooting position - consistently going through the same exact procedures for each attempt - relaxing and optimizing emotions - thinking about the shooting motion - feeling the shooting motion - paying attention to the holding position and the finger placement on the ball - expecting to make the shot - visualizing the hand releasing the ball perfectly, the pathway of ball spinning in the air, the shooting motion, and the ball going through the net	Steps 1 and 2: readying and imaging

II	focusing attention	- focusing on the front area of the rim
		- thinking only of this zone of the rim
		- blocking out internal thoughts, such as "I hope I won't miss the shot"; "I wish somebody else could have taken the shot"; "I need more time for improving my shooting ability"
		- blocking out external distractors, such as
		  * noise
		  * "trash talk" of opponent players standing next to the shooting line
		- executing with a quiet mind
			Step 3: focusing attention

III	evaluating	- looking to see if the ball goes in or if it misses the target - determining why it missed, if it did - paying attention to the follow-through position of the shooting hand - assessing the shooting technique - judging the implementation of the readying, imaging, and focusing attention stages	Step 5: evaluating

Table 2. Case 1 — Free-throw performance in basketball

Phase	Psychological Foundation	Guidelines	5-SA
I	readying (mechanical, mental, and emotional)	- placing the ball on the kicking spot - taking a few steps toward the center of the field - getting into a comfortable position - standing a few seconds; breathing deeply; looking at the center of the goal - looking down; looking up at the goal keeper - starting to move toward the ball - developing consistency in these acts - relaxing - thinking about the kicking motion - feeling the kicking motion - paying attention to the distance between the ball and the body - expecting to make the kick - visualizing the pathway of the ball spinning in the air; the ball going through the goal; and the kicking motion, with the leg kicking the ball perfectly	Steps 1 and 2: readying and imaging
II	focusing attention	- focusing on the central zone of the goal - thinking only of this zone of the goal - blocking out internal thoughts, such as "I hope I won't miss the kick"; "I wish somebody else could have taken the kick"; "I need more time for improving my kicking ability" - blocking out external distractions, such as * noise * goal keeper's distractions - executing with a quiet mind	Step 3: focusing attention
III	evaluating	- this phase may not be applied by the kicker. In most cases, the player performs only one attempt of the penalty kick. It is very unusual to be provided with one more attempt during the game. Thus, the evaluation process should be conducted after the game. It is recommended that the player and the coach observe the kicking performances on the TV screen after they have been videotaped. The player and the coach should examine both the technique and the outcome of the kicking act. This postgame analysis should aid the player in enhancing the development of preperformance routines	Step 5: evaluating

Table 3. Case 2 — An 11-meter kick in soccer

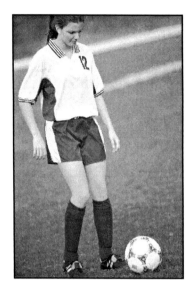

In order to decide what type of guidance to give a player, you must carefully examine the problem and its causes.

In Case 2, Laurie seems to misunderstand how to focus attention on one relevant cue of her kicking performance. She should be guided on how to stay in focus before and during the kicking act. She would probably most benefit from the guidelines presented in the second phase of the preparatory ritual, focusing attention.

The guidelines in Table 3, previous page, can be used in Laurie's case. All are applied to a penalty-kick performance in soccer.

General and specific guidelines should be used by the coach or instructor when presenting a new movement skill to learners. To assist in implementing the guidelines of learning strategies for the effective development of preperformance routines, the following practical recommendations are presented.

Practical Recommendations for the Coach

Effective learning strategies should enhance not only the learning of a movement skill, as has been strongly indicated in the literature (Lidor, 1999; Singer, 2001), but also the development of meaningful preperformance routines. If a learning strategy like the 5-SA is introduced early in the learning process along with the technical knowledge about the movement skill, more beneficial long-term gains should be realized.

The following recommendations may assist the coach or teacher in how to incorporate learning strategies for the development of preperformance routines in any instructional program involving self-paced tasks in team sports, such as ballgame activities. They should

1. Emphasize the mental/psychological aspects of the preperformance routine as much as the physical/mechanical aspects;
2. Integrate the guidelines for the routine along with the technical sport act, implementing such information as early as possible in the learning process; use videotaped modeling to introduce the strategy (see Bouchard and Singer's 1998 field study);
3. Introduce each phase of the routine, such as proposed with the 5-SA, readiness (mechanical, mental, and emotional), focusing attention, and evaluating, one at a time;
4. Emphasize the contribution of each phase of the routine to the actual learning and performing of the skill;
5. Evaluate frequently the effectiveness of the routine;
6. Encourage the development of a consistent routine.

An attempt was made in this chapter to examine developmental and educational considerations of learning strategies, such as the 5-SA, for the establishment of pre- and during-performance routines among beginning learners in ballgame activities. High-level athletes and skilled performers have refined routines that they use so frequently and effectively that they are activated as if they were automatic. These routines should be taught to young people at an early stage of learning in order to be most effective for immediate and long-term success in the execution of any self-paced motor skill.

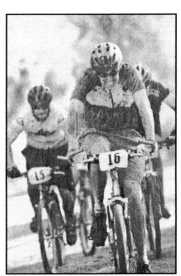

Experienced athletes learn to pinpoint the routine that works and do it the same way in every race.

References

Abernethy, B. (1988). Visual search in sport and ergonomics: Its relationship to selective attention and performer expertise. *Human Performance, 1,* 205-235.

Anderson, A. (1997). Learning strategies in physical education: Self-talk, imagery, and goal-setting. *Journal of Physical Education, Recreation, and Dance, 68(1),* 30-35.

Anderson, J. R. (1990). *Cognitive psychology and its implications* (3rd ed.). New York: W. H. Freeman and Company.

Bandura, A. (1997). *Self-efficacy: The exercise of control.* New York: W. H. Freeman and Company.

Bird, L. (1986). *Bird on basketball.* Reading, MA: Addison-Wesley Publishing Company.

Bouchard, L. J., & Singer, R. N. (1998). Effects of the five-step strategy with videotape modeling on performance of the tennis serve. *Perceptual and Motor Skills, 86,* 739-746.

Boutcher, S. H., & Zinsser, N. W. (1990). Cardiac deceleration of elite and beginning golfers during putting. *Journal of Sport and Exercise Psychology, 12,* 37-47.

Carver, C. S., & Scheier, M. F. (1998). *On the self-regulation of behavior.* Cambridge, UK: Cambridge University Press.

Chen, D., & Singer, R. N. (1992). Self-regulation and cognitive strategies in sport participation. *International Journal of Sport Psychology, 23,* 277-300.

Christina, R. W., & Corcos, D. M. (1988). *Coaches' guide to teaching sport skills.* Champaign, IL: Human Kinetics.

Clark, F. J., & Norch, K. W. (1986). Kinesthesia. In K. R. Boff, L. Kaufman, & J. P. Thomas (Eds.), *Handbook of perception and performance* (pp.1-62). New York: Wiley.

Cohn, P. J. (1990). Preperformance routines in sport: Theoretical support and practical applications. *The Sport Psychologist, 4,* 301-312.

Crews, D. J. (1993). Self-regulation strategies in sport and exercise. In R. N. Singer, M. Murphey, & L. K. Tennant (Eds.), *Handbook of research on sport psychology* (pp. 557-568). New York: Macmillan.

Frehlich, S. G. (1997). *Quiet eye duration as an index of cognitive processing: The effect of task complexity and task duration on visual search patterns and performance in highly-skilled and lesser-skilled billiards players.* Unpublished doctoral dissertation, University of Florida, Gainesville.

Gallagher, J. D., & Thomas, J. R. (1986). Developmental effects of grouping and recoding on learning a movement series. *Research Quarterly for Exercise and Sport, 57,* 117-127.

Gardner, H. (1983). *Frames of mind: The theory of multiple intelligence.* New York: Basic Books.

Gould, D., & Udry, E. (1994). Psychological skills for enhancing performance: Arousal regulation strategies. *Medicine and Science in Sports and Exercise, 26,* 478-485.

Hall, E. G., & Erffmeyer, E. S. (1983). The effect of visuo-motor behavior rehearsal with videotaped modeling on free throw accuracy of intercollegiate female basketball players. *Journal of Sport Psychology, 5,* 343-346.

Hardy, L., & Nelson, D. (1988). Self-regulation training in sport and work. *Ergonomics, 31,* 1573-1583.

Hatfield, B. D., Landers, D. L., & Ray, W. J. (1984). Cognitive processes during self-paced motor performance: An electroencephalographic profile of skilled marksmen. *Journal of Sport Psychology, 6,* 42-59.

Hatfield, B. D., Landers, D. L., & Ray, W. J. (1987). Cardiovascular-CNS interactions during a self-paced, intentional state: Elite marksmanship performance. *Psychophysiology, 24,* 542-549.

Henry, F. M., & Rogers, D. E. (1960). Increased response latency for complicated movements and a "memory drum" theory of neuromotor reaction. *Research Quarterly, 41,* 448-458.

Jordan, M. (1994). *I can't accept not trying.* San Francisco: Harper San Francisco.

Lacey, J. I. (1967). Somatic response patterning and stress: Some revisions of activation theory. In M. H. Appley & R. Trumbull (Eds.), *Psychological stress* (pp. 14-42). New York: Appleton-Century Croft.

Lamirand, M., & Rainey, D. (1994). Mental imagery, relaxation, and accuracy of basketball foul shooting. *Perceptual and Motor Skills, 78,* 1229-1230.

Landers, D. M., Han, M., Salazare, W., Petruzzello, S. J., Kubitz, K. A., & Gannon, T. L. (1994). Effects of learning on electroencephalographic and electrocardiographic patterns in novice archers. *International Journal of Sport Psychology, 25,* 313-330.

Lee, T. D., Chamberlin, C. G., & Hodges, N. J. (2001). Practice. In R. N. Singer, H. A. Hausenblas, & C. M. Janelle (Eds.), *Handbook of sport psychology* (2nd ed., pp. 115-143). New York: Wiley.

Lidor, R. (1997). Effectiveness of a structured learning strategy on acquisition of game-related gross motor tasks in school settings. *Perceptual and Motor Skills, 84,* 67-80.

Lidor, R. (1999). Learning strategies and the enhancement of self-paced motor tasks: Theoretical and practical implications. In R. Lidor & M. Bar-Eli (Eds.), *Sport psychology: Linking theory and practice* (pp. 109-132). Morgantown, WV: Fitness Information Technology.

Lidor, R., Arnon, M., & Bronstein, A. (1999). The effectiveness of a learning (cognitive) strategy on free throw performances in basketball. *Applied Research in Coaching and Athletics Annual, 14,* 59-72.

Lidor, R., Tennant, K. L., & Singer, R. N. (1996). The generalizability effect of three learning strategies across motor task performances. *International Journal of Sport Psychology, 27,* 22-36.

Lobmeyer, D. L., & Wasserman, E. A. (1986). Preliminaries to free throw shooting: Superstitious behavior? *Journal of Sport Behavior, 9,* 70-78.

Logan, G. D. (1988). Automaticity, resources, and memory: Theoretical controversies and practical implications. *Human Factors, 30,* 583-598.

Louganis, G. (1995). *Breaking the surface.* New York: Random House.

McPherson, S. L. (1993). The influence of player experience on problem solving during batting preparation in baseball. *Journal of Sport and Exercise Psychology, 15,* 304-325.

Moran, A. P. (1996). *The psychology of concentration in sport performers: A cognitive analysis.* East Sussex, UK: Psychology Press.

Nevett, M. E., & French, K. E. (1997). The development of sport specific planning, rehearsal, and updating of plans during defensive youth baseball game performance. *Research Quarterly for Exercise and Sport, 68,* 203-214.

Perkins, D. (1992). *Smart schools - from training memories to educating minds.* New York: Cambridge University Press.

Radlo, S. J. (1997). *The effectiveness of Singer's five-step strategy during a competitive situation: A behavioral and psychophysiological investigation.* Unpublished doctoral dissertation, University of Florida, Gainesville.

Radlo, S. J., Steinberg, G. M., Singer, R. N., Barba, D. A., & Melnikov, A. (2002). The influence of an attentional focus strategy on alpha brain wave activity, heart rate, and dart-throwing performances. *International Journal of Sport Psychology, 33,* 205-217.

Salazar, W., Landers, D. M., Petruzzello, S. J., Crews, D. J., Kubits, K. A., & Han, M. (1990). Hemispheric asymmetry, cardiac response, and performance in elite archers. *Research Quarterly in Exercise and Sport, 61,* 351-359.

Schmidt, R. A., & Lee, T. D. (1999). *Motor control and learning: A behavioral emphasis* (3rd ed.). Champaign, IL: Human Kinetics.

Schmidt, R. A., & Wrisberg, C. A. (2000). *Motor learning and performance: A problem-based learning approach* (2nd ed.). Champaign, IL: Human Kinetics.

Schnieder, W., & Shiffrin, R. (1977). Controlled and automatic human information processing: I. Detection search, and attention. *Psychological Review, 84,* 1-66.

Singer, R. N. (1978). Motor skills and learner strategies. In H. F. O'Neil (Ed.), *Learning strategies* (pp. 79-106). New York: Academic Press.

Singer, R. N. (1980). *Motor learning and human performance* (3rd ed.). New York: Macmillan.

Singer, R. N. (1986). Children in physical activity: Motor learning considerations. In G. A. Stull & H. M. Eckert (Eds.), *The Academy papers: Effects of physical activity on children* (pp. 64-74). Champaign, IL: Human Kinetics.

Singer, R. N. (1988). Strategies and metastrategies in learning and performing self-paced athletic skills. *The Sport Psychologist, 2,* 49-68.

Singer, R. N. (2001). Performance and human factors: Considerations about cognition and attention for self-paced and externally-paced events. *Ergonomics, 43,* 1661-1680.

Singer, R. N., & Chen, D. (1994). A classification scheme for cognitive strategies: Implications for learning and teaching psychomotor skills. *Research Quarterly for Exercise and Sport, 65,* 143-151.

Singer, R. N., & Gershon, R. F. (1979). Learning strategies, cognitive processes, and motor learning. In H. F. O'Neil & C. D. Spielberger (Eds.), *Cognitive and affective learning strategies* (pp. 215-248). New York: Academic Press.

Singer, R. N., Hausenblas, H. A., & Janelle, C. M. (Eds.) (2001). *Handbook of sport psychology* (2nd ed.). New York: Wiley.

Singer, R. N., Lidor, R., & Cauraugh, J. H. (1993). To be aware or not aware? What to think about while learning and performing a motor skill. *The Sport Psychologist, 7,* 19-30.

Singer, R. N., Lidor, R., & Cauraugh, J. H. (1994). Focus of attention during motor skill performance. *Journal of Sports Sciences, 12,* 335-340.

Singer, R. N., Murphey, M., & Tennant, L. K. (Eds.) (1993). *Handbook of research on sport psychology.* New York: Macmillan.

Southard, D., & Miracle, A. (1993). Rhythmicity, ritual, and motor performance: A study of free throw shooting in basketball. *Research Quarterly for Exercise and Sport, 64,* 284-290.

Southard, D., Miracle, A., & Landwer, G. (1989). Ritual and free-throw shooting in basketball. *Journal of Sports Sciences, 7,* 163-173.

Sternberg, R. J. (1985). *Beyond IQ: A triarchic theory of human intelligence.* New York: Cambridge University Press.

Vickers, J. N. (1992). Gaze control in putting. *Perception, 21,* 117-132.

Vickers, J. N. (1996). Visual control when aiming at a far target. *Journal of Experimental Psychology: Human Perception and Performance, 22,* 342-354.

Vickers, J. N. (1997). Control of visual attention during the basketball free throw. *The American Journal of Sports Medicine, 24,* 93-97.

Weinberg, R. S., & Gould, D. (1999). *Foundations of sport and exercise psychology* (2nd ed.). Champaign, IL: Human Kinetics.

Weinstein, C. E., & Mayer, R. A. (1986). The teaching of learning strategies. In M.C. Wittrock (Ed.), *Handbook of research on teaching* (pp. 315-327). New York: Macmillan.

Wrisberg, C. A., & Anshel, M. H. (1989). The effect of cognitive strategies on free throw shooting performance of young athletes. *The Sport Psychologist, 3,* 95-104.

Wrisberg, C. A., & Pain, R. L. (1992). The preshot interval and free throw shooting accuracy: An exploratory investigation. *The Sport Psychologist, 6,* 14-23.

CHAPTER 5

The Principles of Team Building and Their Application to Sport Teams

Paul A. Estabrooks and Paul W. Dennis

Abstract

The following chapter has been designed to provide the reader with practical team-building intervention strategies that have been developed utilizing a strong theoretical basis. In order to realize this objective, our chapter outlines the nature of groups. Specifically, the conditions necessary to consider a "collective of individuals" as "a group" are delineated. Group cohesion is described and defined in terms of its dynamic and multidimensional nature, and a brief review of the empirical evidence associated with cohesion and sport is provided. Finally, the reader is provided with step-by-step instructions regarding the implementation of both direct and indirect team-building interventions.

"I always taught players that the main ingredient of stardom is the rest of the team. It's amazing how much can be accomplished when no one gets the credit" (Cypert, 1991, p. 180). These were the words of John Wooden, one of the winningest coaches in United States college basketball history. Clearly Coach Wooden was alluding to the oft believed dictum that united we stand, divided we fall. Consequently, the necessity of developing team harmony amongst team members has become an important priority for practitioners in the team sport setting. Coaches in particular seek ways to build an effective team. Research on group dynamics outlines that the cohesive nature of the group developed around both social and task-specific interactions may be essential for team effectiveness (Carron & Hausenblas, 1998). Unfortunately, many coaches struggle to find a systematic program to develop a strong sense of cohesion within their teams. It is not enough for the coach to proclaim the traditional "there is no 'I' in team." In fact, such lip service is often ineffective and occasionally even laughable.

The main purpose of this chapter is to outline systematic procedures to develop a strong sense of team cohesion. To achieve this purpose we will (a) outline the nature of groups, (b) define and describe group cohesion, (c) review the empirical evidence regarding the effects of strong team cohesion, and (d) outline systematic team-building interventions (direct and indirect) to develop team cohesion.

The Nature of Groups

Prior to using a group dynamics intervention such as team building, it is necessary to understand what makes up a group. Zander (1982) noted that an important distinction must be made between a group and a collection of individuals. He identified ten characteristics that differentiate a group from a collection of individuals. People in groups

1. talk freely,
2. are interested in the welfare of the collective as a whole,
3. feel that their associates are helpful,
4. try to assist those associates,
5. refer to the collection of individuals as "we" and to other collections as "they,"
6. faithfully participate in group activities,
7. are not primarily interested in individual accomplishments,
8. are concerned with the activities of other members,
9. do not see others as rivals, and
10. are not often absent.

Similarly, Carron (1993) noted that some of the more salient features of groups are a collective identity, a sense of shared purpose, structured patterns of interaction and communication, personal and task interdependence, interpersonal attraction, a shared common fate, and a perception of the unit as a collective. Based upon the above criteria, it is clear that a sport team may be considered a group. Because sport teams are able to demonstrate these characteristics and are clearly groups, it is appropriate to apply the principles of group dynamics to ensure a more effective team.

Group Cohesion

Groups become more effective when they maximize the importance of the collective and minimize the importance of each individual. The relative importance of the collective and the individual within the collective can be developed and reinforced by a strong sense of group cohesion. Cohesion may be defined as "a dynamic process that is reflected in the tendency for a group to stick together and remain united in the pursuit of its instrumental objectives and/or for the satisfaction of member affective needs" (Carron, Brawley, & Widmeyer, 1998, p. 213). Cohesion is associated with four main properties. It is multidimensional, dynamic, instrumental, and affective. First, cohesion is multidimensional in that there are many factors that cause a group to stick together. Thus, a team may be united around task objectives, social objectives, or both. It is conceivable that a team may develop strong cohesion around the group task yet be in open conflict from a social perspective. Second, cohesion is a dynamic process and as such, it changes over time. For example, performance has been consistently related to cohesion, both as an antecedent and an outcome. Therefore, a basketball team could have very high cohesion after winning the first three games of the season; however if the same team were to lose the next three games, the cohesive nature of the team might decrease. Third, cohesion is instrumental or purposeful. In volleyball, task cohesion is developed with the purpose of allowing the team to bump, set, and spike the ball over the net, whereas social cohesion is developed to afford the team members social support and satisfaction. Forth, cohesion has an affective dimension. Satisfaction and a sense of belonging are affective outcomes associated with a highly cohesive group.

Now that the coach or practitioner understands the nature of group cohesion, the next necessary step is to determine how to assess if a team is or is not cohesive. A number of measurement tools have been developed to assess group cohesion (e.g., Sport Cohesiveness Questionnaire, Multidimensional Sport Cohesion Instrument). However, only one inventory was developed based on theory and has resulted in consistently reliable and valid findings. Carron, Widmeyer, and Brawley (1985) designed the Group Environment Questionnaire (GEQ), an instrument that assesses cohesion in sport teams. The GEQ is based on a conceptual framework of group cohesion based on the social cognitions of individual team members. The perceptions that each member holds about the cohesiveness of the group are a reflection of the cohesive nature of the group as a totality. The framework includes four dimensions based on individual attractions and integration to the group around task and social situations. Group integration may be described as the individual's perceptions about the closeness or degree of unification of the group. Often described as "us, our, we" perceptions, an example of a group integration statement is "Our team is united in the pursuit of our goals and objectives." Individual attractions to the group are the individual's perceptions about personal motivations that draw him or her to the group and that are reflected by "I, my, and me" perceptions. An example statement would be "I enjoy the social atmosphere of this group." The need to distinguish between task oriented and socially oriented concerns is also essential. Therefore, task orientation is motivation toward achieving the group's objectives, and social orientation is motivation toward developing social relations. The GEQ has been shown to possess adequate reliability and strong predictive validity (see Carron et al., 1998 for a complete review).

The relationship between perceptions of cohesion and enhanced team dynamics is an important concept for coaches and players to understand. For example, cohesion is an output or product of conditions present in three categories: the group's environment, the group's structure, and the group's processes (Carron, Spink, & Prapavessis, 1997). Specific factors identified for each of the categories include proximity and distinctiveness (group environment); role clarity, role acceptance, leadership, and conformity to group norms (group structure); and cooperation, sacrifice, goals, and objectives (group process).

Based upon previous research efforts (e.g., Carron & Ball, 1977; Carron & Chelladurai, 1981; Dawe & Carron, 1990; Kinal & Carron, 1987; Shangi & Carron, 1987), three conclusions related to the cohesion-performance relationship can be advanced. First, cohesion in sport teams is positively associated with performance success. This relationship is evident in a reciprocal fashion; that is, high group cohesion leads to performance success and continued performance success leads to high group cohesion. Second, the performance-cohesion relationship is stronger than the cohesion-performance relationship. Therefore, although group cohesion improves performance, one of the best interventions for the improvement of cohesion is performance success. This information is invaluable when planning preseason exhibition matches. Arranging opponents who are challenging yet beatable could be an effective component of a cohesion-based intervention strategy. Third, immediate game outcome does not produce changes in cohesiveness. Hence, a single loss or victory will not change the underlying perceptions of cohesion held by team members. Additionally, a recent meta-analysis showed a significant relationship between cohesion and performance (Mullen & Copper, 1994). In fact, if groups were thought of as a continuum from artificial groups (e.g., laboratory experimental groups) to nonsport/nonmilitary real groups to military groups and finally to sports teams, the impact of cohesion becomes more salient along the continuum (Mullen & Copper, 1994).

Although there may be a number of moderating variables that might affect the relative importance of each cohesion dimension, research in the area is relatively sparse. Age and gender have been suggested as moderators of the differential importance of the dimensions of group cohesion; again, no data have been found to support this supposition. However, one may hypothesize that individual motivation may be the primary moderator of group-cohesion dimensions and outcomes. Logically, it may be assumed that adolescents may initially be drawn to the social aspect of a sport to fulfill a need to belong. Conversely, a young adult may not be motivated by the need to belong, but rather by an attraction to a specific task or sport, and thus, choose to participate for task reasons. Having stated that, science has long been a devil's advocate to logic, and as such, we must stress that before any conclusions are made regarding the moderating effect of age and gender, further research is required.

One moderator that does seem to have an impact on the differential importance of the dimensions of cohesion is the level of competition. Carron and his associates (Carron, Widmeyer, & Brawley, 1988) found that level of competition had an impact on the predictive validity of different dimensions of cohesion. Elite athletes who maintained sport involvement were correctly classified 80% of the time by a function that included individual attractions to the group's task and the group integration-task and social components. Conversely, in a sample of recreational athletes, the dimension of group integration-social was the only discriminator of adherence behavior.

Regardless of the moderators of group cohesion, the team-building concepts that will be outlined below should be effective. The efficacy of each of the intervention strategies is based upon determining the underlying motivations of the individual and the collective, and for these reasons, these strategies are appropriate for teams of any level.

Team Building and Cohesion

Newman (1984) noted that team building is designed to "promote an increased sense of unity and cohesiveness and enable the team to function together more smoothly and effectively" (p. 27). More recently, the term team building has been used to describe a method for a team to "(a) increase effectiveness, (b) satisfy the needs of its members, or (c) improve work conditions" (Brawley & Paskevich, 1997, p. 13). At the core of any team-building program is the expectation that the intervention will produce a more cohesive unit (Carron et al., 1997).

The term team building has come to be popularly associated with a range of activities/games designed to build important aspects of the team such as trust, communication, leadership, and ice breaking. A comprehensive description of short games and activities can be found in books such as *The Big Book of Team Building Games* (Newstrom & Scannell, 1998) or Pell's *The Complete Idiot's Guide to Team Building* (2000). However, brief games and activities are of limited utility if they are not complemented by some of the more fundamental team-building strategies.

Four primary methods that have been used in recent years to increase team cohesion and ultimately effectiveness are goal setting, interpersonal relations, role expectations, and the managerial grid. The goal-setting method emphasizes the importance of establishing goals and objectives so the group may function more effectively. The interpersonal-relations method seeks to minimize internal conflicts amongst group members. The role-expectations method is used to clarify roles and obligations of the group. Finally, the managerial grid is an approach that considers the person and the product in the team-building process.

There are two approaches used for implementation of these interventions—a direct and an indirect approach. The direct approach has the sport psychologist/facilitator work directly with the team employing a hands-on approach to team building. Conversely, the indirect approach has the coach act as the agent through which the team-building intervention is presented to the group.

Coaches may be reluctant to acquiesce to the direct approach for two reasons. First, the coach would have to relinquish part of his or her control over the team members to the facilitator. Second, some coaches may believe that the sport psychologist/facilitator may be using the team to promote personal interests. Nevertheless, coaches who lack the knowledge to implement the techniques used to promote team cohesion would be wise to solicit the advice of a facilitator. We will use team-building interventions developed around group goal setting and interpersonal relations to illustrate an indirect and a direct approach, respectively.

Strategies for Developing Team Cohesion in Team Ball Activities

Team Goal Setting

Goal setting is a universal phenomenon designed to assist athletes by (a) directing their attention toward a particular task, (b) mobilizing their effort, (c) increasing their ability to prolong persistence to effort, and (d) developing and implementing new learning strategies (Locke & Latham, 1985). In general, the goal-setting research indicates that challenging goals enhance motivation and performance (Locke, Shaw, Saari, & Latham, 1981). Moreover, goals have been demonstrated to be powerful motivators because they provide standards from which to evaluate continuous performances. As a result, the motivational factor in goal setting can be viewed as the attainment of a desired goal or standard (George & Feltz, 1995).

One important characteristic of team goal setting is member participation. It should be emphasized that group goal setting is more advantageous than individual goal setting, and the more people that participate, the greater the sense of ownership. For example, Widmeyer and Ducharme (1997) noted that having a team goal and team participation in that goal has been demonstrated to enhance task cohesion of athletic teams. Moreover, Brawley, Carron, and Widmeyer (1993) found that the group variable cohesion was "(a) related to the psychological consequence of team satisfaction with group goals, and (b) greater among those individuals who perceive that their team engages in group goal setting for competition" (p. 257).

A related point is the benefit of indirectly applying the intervention through the coach. One of the more salient features of the indirect approach is the notion that the coach is often viewed as the primary arbitrator of group goals, individual roles, and leadership style (Carron et al., 1997). As a result, coaches may take greater ownership in presenting the intervention. In addition, there may be an expectation by the team to have their coach engaged in initiatives that are thought to be an integral component to enhancing team effectiveness.

Widmeyer and McGuire (1996) developed a four-phase team-building intervention through goal setting that consisted of an educational phase, a goal-development phase, an implementation phase, and a renewal phase. Although the intervention was developed for elite ice hockey teams, there is applicability to team ball activities as well. The following then is a four-phase, indirect team-building intervention through goal setting adopted from Widmeyer and McGuire (1996) for basketball.

The educational phase. The educational phase is conducted at the beginning of the basketball season. During this phase, the coach reviews several principles underlying the importance of goal setting, team building, and cohesion with the members of the basketball team. For example, during the presentation, the coach highlights the relationship between perceptions of cohesiveness and improved team dynamics. Also, the coach briefly describes the ways in which goal setting works and the importance of player participation in collective goal setting. In addition, the coach emphasizes that team goals and process goals are more important to the development of greater harmony than outcome goals are. In short, the purpose of the educational phase is to promote the notion that goal setting, from a team perspective, increases the chance for greater team effectiveness more than individual goal setting or no goal setting at all does.

Concept	Benefit	Strategy
Team building	Improve team effectiveness	Discussion with players regarding the importance of stressing "we" versus "I"
Brief overview of group cohesion reflects the tendency of the group to stick together and remain united	Improved team dynamics (e.g., cohesion group process factors including cooperation and sacrifice)	Potluck team dinner for players, coaches, and support staff celebrated by means of serving each other (e.g., team captain asks a teammate, "May I get you a plate of pasta and chicken?") Group members must not prepare a plate for themselves
Team goal setting	Influence team cohesion by providing a team focus	The coach asks the members of the team to identify what the team focus should be for the current season

Table 1. Team building through goal setting in team ball activities educational phase

Table 1 contains an example of concepts and activities to be presented during the education phase. As previously indicated, cooperation and sacrifice have been identified as specific factors to be emphasized during team-building exercises. Thus, one strategy designed to emphasize the importance of cooperation and sacrifice is a team dinner, whereby the players, coaches, and support staff are engaged in a potluck sit-down meal. However, no one is permitted to serve him- or herself. The coach must stipulate that the idea of the team dinner is to ask each other, "What can I get you to eat/drink?"

The goal-development phase. After the team meal, the goal-development phase has the coach ask the team members to identify performance measures as they pertain to basketball (see Table 2). For example, factors such as foul shooting, field goals, layups, blocked shots, assists, and forced turnovers are mentioned. The coach then asks each team member to select the performance measures that he or she considers most important for team success. The next step is to have the athletes form small groups to discuss their choices and to decide on a consensus for their small group. The team then reconvenes in an attempt to establish a consensus of the most important performance measures deemed critical for team success.

Offensive Play	Defensive Play
1. Assists	1. Blocked shots
2. Field goals	2. Forced turnovers
3. Free throws	3. Jump shots
4. Layups	4. Rebounds
5. Rebounds	5. Steals

Table 2. Potential performance measures for basketball

Upon identifying the team's most important performance measures, it is recommended that the process be repeated to determine the appropriate level for the goal for an upcoming five-game segment. For example, the coach, using the previous year's statistics as a guide (e.g., free-throw shooting percentages), asks the team members to independently arrive at a goal. Using the same protocol listed above, consensus is then achieved in a small group setting, followed by a discussion amongst the entire team. Once identification of the group goals is complete, it is important that the team coach or captain outline the appropriate steps necessary to achieve the stated goal. For example, if the team has identified a goal of 85% foul shooting accuracy, the coach/captain should outline mechanisms by which this goal should be obtained (i.e., everyone shoots 100 free throws a day).

The implementation phase. The implementation phase is designed to have an assistant coach, or the team's statistician, record the team's performance and compare it to the predetermined performance measures. In other words, if the team has set a goal of 85% foul shooting accuracy, the performance toward that particular goal would be monitored.

The renewal phase. As previously mentioned, the level for each team goal is determined for five-game segments. Based upon the team's progress toward achieving the identified goals, the players may revise the goals for the next five-game segment based upon the feedback from monitoring the team's accomplishments. In short, the coach may ask the athletes to reconsider their goals as a group and set new ones.

In summary, research has suggested that group goals enhance performance as effectively as individual goals (Locke & Latham, 1990). Moreover, the more cohesive the team is, the more motivated the athletes will be to strive to reach their goals. The team goal-setting strategy outlined above is designed to identify the performance measures deemed by the team to be critical for success. Because there is a greater sense of ownership amongst the team members in this intervention, it is hoped that the effort and persistence generated by the team as a whole will lead to greater success.

An Interpersonal Relations Approach

Crace and Hardy (1997) have introduced a model that focuses on a values-based approach using the practitioner as the direct administrator of the intervention. The rationale for the Crace and Hardy (1997) model is that by assessing values, there will be greater potential to enhance team chemistry. The steps associated with the model focus on (a) understanding each other from a values perspective, (b) understanding the predominant values of the team, (c) identifying the factors that promote and interfere with cohesion from a values perspective, and (e) developing strategies to improve mutual respect and subsequent cohesion.

Clearly, the basis of the Crace and Hardy (1997) intervention model is the values of both the individual and the collective; therefore, prior to implementation of the intervention, an assessment of team member values is necessary.

This assessment can be accommodated by the administration of the Life Values Inventory (Crace & Brown, 1996). The Life Values Inventory uses both qualitative and quantitative components to assist individuals in rating and ranking their values (Crace & Hardy, 1997). The quantitative component comprises 14 scales made up of three items each. They include achievement, belonging, concern for the environment, concern for others, creativity, health and activity, humility, independence, loyalty to family or group, privacy, prosperity, responsibility, scientific understanding, and spirituality. The respondents rank each item based upon the degree to which the value guides their individual behavior. The qualitative component of the inventory is used to further illustrate the priority of individual values through open-ended questions such as "Who do you admire most?," "If you won a lottery, what would you do with the money?," and "Do you have a motto?" Although the Life Values Inventory is relatively new and lacking in reliability and validity data, there are four generalizations that promote its use (Crace & Hardy, 1997). First, it was developed based on extensive research into cultural values. Second, it is a brief inventory with sound internal consistency (quantitative component). Third, the use of a qualitative component enhances the depth of understanding for the sport psychology practitioner. Fourth, it uses a holistic approach assessing all major life roles simultaneously.

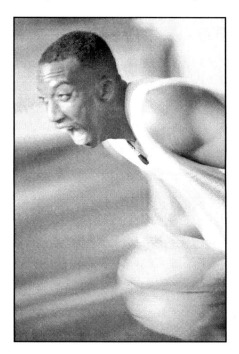

One integral aspect of the intervention model is the integration of individual needs with team goals.

Step	Concept	Activity
1	Demonstrate the importance of individual differences	The team facilitator lectures to coaches and players concerning the principles of team-building strategies.
2	Understanding individual differences	Athletes are instructed to write three important goals they have for themselves. Small groups are formed to discuss answers.
3	Understanding the interaction of values and life roles	Athletes select 4-6 major roles that currently demand time and energy.
4	Predominant characteristics of the team	Athletes discuss how a major part of success on the team will be determined by how well the team values are satisfied.
5	Factors that promote and interfere with team cohesion	Athletes discuss the strengths and challenges of the team profile.
6	Action plan for mutual respect	Athletes brainstorm strategies to facilitate attainment of team values.
7	Coaches learn to understand what the team experienced	The facilitator takes the coaches through some exercises to clarify their values and life roles.
8	Follow-up and evaluation	The facilitator schedules meetings with the coaches and team to discuss the effectiveness of the team-building program.

Table 3. Summary of the values-based direct approach advanced by Crace and Hardy (1997)

Once the assessment of values is complete, the values-based intervention model follows eight steps, as can be seen in Table 3. Briefly, during Step 1, the facilitator introduces the coaches and players to the principles behind team building. The emphasis is on team synergy whereby differing personalities blend to achieve a common goal. For example, the facilitator would acknowledge that although individuals are different on a basketball team, learning how to strive toward a common goal is a necessary ingredient to becoming an effective team. Step 2 focuses on understanding individual differences. For example, on a basketball team, the facilitator instructs athletes to write three important goals they have for themselves within a specified time frame. Upon completing the task, they form small groups and discuss their answers. The group reconvenes and each athlete shares two answers from his or her partner that the athlete found most interesting. In Step 3, athletes list up to three values they hope to have satisfied within a particular role. For example, an athlete may hope to have achievement satisfied in his or her role. Step 4 focuses on the predominant values. The facilitator records the most important values listed by athletes on a board and conducts a frequency count as they are identified. The five values with the most number of responses are the top team values. Step 5 provides an opportunity for players to discuss the strengths and challenges of the team profile based upon the top team values. Step 6 includes a brainstorming session whereby ideas are shared in an attempt to facilitate the attainment of team values. As a consequence of the discussion in Step 6, the facilitator may be required to educate the team on specific mental skills (e.g., stress management or goal setting). Step 7 has the facilitator work with the coaches to clarify their values and life roles. Step 8 requires follow-up and evaluation to discuss the effectiveness of the program.

Summary

A popular tenet advanced by coaches in sport situations is the importance of synergistic teamwork whereby the strengths and talents of individuals are molded together so that they may become greater than the sum of their parts. Thus, developing team cohesion to enhance team dynamics is an essential concept for practitioners, coaches, athletes, and support staff to understand. Developing team cohesion can be accomplished through the use of an effective team-building program. There are two approaches used in an attempt to accomplish this. The indirect approach has the coach act as the agent through which the team-building intervention is proposed to the group, whereas the direct approach has an individual outside the team (the sport psychologist/facilitator) work with the team throughout the course of the season. Team-building approaches that use goal setting, for example, attempt to motivate group members to be more goal and objectives oriented. On the other hand, a values-based approach is used to enhance team chemistry by focusing on interpersonal relations, such as the core beliefs that guide behavior. In short, team-building interventions that emphasize the "collective good" are viewed as strategies that increase the likelihood of enhancing group processes and team cohesion.

References

Brawley, L. R., Carron, A. V., & Widmeyer, W. N. (1993). The influence of the group and its cohesiveness on perceptions of group goal-related variables. *Journal of Sport and Exercise Psychology, 15,* 245-260.

Brawley, L. R., & Paskevich, D. M. (1997). Conducting team building research in the context of sport and exercise. *Journal of Applied Sport Psychology, 9,* 11-40.

Carron, A. V. (1993). The sport team as an effective group. In J. Williams (Ed.), *Applied sport psychology: Personal growth to peak performance* (pp. 110-121). Mountain View, CA: Mayfield Publishing.

Carron, A. V., & Ball, J. R. (1977). Cause-effect characteristics of cohesiveness and participation motivation in intercollegiate hockey. *International Review of Sport Sociology, 12,* 49-60.

Carron, A. V., Brawley, L. R., & Widmeyer, W. N. (1998). The measurement of cohesiveness in sport groups. In J. L. Duda (Ed.), *Advancements in sport and exercise psychology measurement* (pp. 213-226). Morgantown, WV: Fitness Information Technology.

Carron, A. V., & Chelladurai, P. (1981). The dynamics of group cohesion in sport. *Journal of Sport Psychology, 3,* 123-139.

Carron, A. V., & Hausenblas, H. A. (1998). *Group dynamics in sport* (2nd ed.). Morgantown, WV: Fitness Information Technology.

Carron, A. V., Spink, K. S., & Prapavessis, H. (1997). Team building and cohesiveness in the sport and exercise setting: Use of indirect interventions. *Journal of Applied Sport Psychology, 9,* 61-72.

Carron, A. V., Widmeyer, W. N., & Brawley, L. R. (1985). The development of an instrument to assess cohesion in sport teams: The Group Environment Questionnaire. *Journal of Sport Psychology, 7,* 244-266.

Carron, A. V., Widmeyer, W. N., & Brawley, L. R. (1988). Group cohesion and individual adherence to physical activity. *Journal of Sport and Exercise Psychology, 10,* 127-138.

Crace, R. K., & Brown, D. (1996). *Life Values Inventory.* Chapel Hill, NC: Life Values Resources.

Crace, R. K., & Hardy, C. J. (1997). Individual values and the team building process. *Journal of Applied Sport Psychology, 9,* 41-60.

Cypert, S.A. (1991). *Believe and achieve: W. Clement Stone's 17 principles of success.* New York: Avon Press.

Dawe, S., & Carron, A. V. (1990, October). *Interrelationships among role accept-ance, role clarity, task cohesion, and social cohesion.* Paper presented at the Canadian Psychomotor Learning and Sport Psychology Conference, Windsor, Ontario.

George, T. R., & Feltz, D. L. (1995). Motivation in sport from a collective effica-cy perspective. *International Journal of Sport Psychology, 26,* 98-116.

Kinal, S., & Carron, A. V. (1987). Effects of game outcome on cohesion in male and female intercollegiate teams. *Canadian Journal of Sport Sciences, 12,* 12.

Locke, E. A., & Latham, G. P. (1985). The application of goal setting to sports. *Journal of Sport Psychology, 7,* 205-222.

Locke, E. A., & Latham, G. P. (1990). *A theory of goal setting and task motivation.* Englewood Cliffs, NJ: Prentice-Hall.

Locke, E. A., Shaw, K. N., Saari, L. M., & Latham, G. P. (1981). Goal setting and task performance. *Psychological Bulletin, 90,* 125-152.

Mullen, B., & Copper, C. (1994). The relation between group cohesiveness and performance: An integration. *Psychological Bulletin, 115,* 210-227.

Newman, B. (1984). Expediency as benefactor: How team building saves time and gets the job done. *Training and Development Journal, 38,* 26-30.

Newstrom, J., & Scannell, E. (1998). *The big book of team building games: Trust-building activities, team spirit exercises, and other fun things to do.* New York: McGraw-Hill.

Pell, A. R. (2000). *The complete idiot's guide to team building.* Indianapolis, IN: MacMillan.

Shangi, G., & Carron, A. V. (1987). Group cohesion and its relationship with per-formance satisfaction among high school basketball players. *Canadian Journal of Sport Sciences, 12,* 20.

Widmeyer, W. N., & Ducharme, K. (1997). Team building through team goal set-ting. *Journal of Applied Sport Psychology, 9,* 97-113.

Widmeyer, W. N., & McGuire, E. J. (1996, May). *Sport psychology for ice hockey. Presentation to Ontario Intermediate Coaching Clinic,* Waterloo, Ontario.

Zander, A. (1982). *Making groups effective.* San Francisco: Jossey-Bass.

CHAPTER 6

Understanding and Managing Emotions in Team Sports

Cal Botterill and Tom Patrick

Abstract

Much attention has been given to an appreciation and understanding of the relationship between emotions and performance in sport. Of importance to athletes, coaches, and sport scientists is achieving an improved understanding of how emotions affect performance and how they can be managed more effectively. This chapter presents a general discussion of emotion in sport derived primarily from the literature within sport psychology. As well, the authors' collective practical experiences through their work with elite athletes and coaches in Canada are discussed. Important emotions are described and practical implications outlined. Finally, suggestions for improving emotional preparation and emotional management are provided as they relate to optimizing performance in team sport.

Few would argue that sport is one of the most emotional fields in life. The roles that passion and emotion play in individual and team sport are formidable. With team sport, however, the effects of emotion are exponentially expanded. The interactive emotional dynamics between teammates and opponents make for powerful drama and tremendous tests of emotional readiness, team solidarity, and commitment.

The old sport adage "you need everyone in big games" is even more important when we consider the emotional contribution of every player. Each individual affects the emotional climate and the "depth" of belief, so "role" players can be every bit as important as (if not more important than) "star" players. Despite the rhetoric on passion and emotions, however, very little has been written to help us understand this domain.

Although research does exist regarding mood and performance (Crocker, Alderman, & Smith, 1988; Hanin & Syrja, 1995; Prapavessis & Grove, 1991), some research has been unable to establish mood as a predictor for performance (Hassmen & Blomstrand, 1995). It has been suggested that further research must be conducted to better understand how mood fluctuations affect athletic performance (Terry, 1995). In addition, most research does not provide information regarding the importance of, or management strategies for, the construct of emotion. Goleman's book *Emotional Intelligence* (1995) begins to sensitize one to the critical issues long overlooked in this domain. In sport, we have had a lot of experience with emotion, and our best insights need to be documented and shared.

Lazarus (2000) has recently attempted to apply his cognitive-motivational-relational theory of emotion to an understanding of performance in competitive sports. He identified 15 discrete emotions that are likely implicated and provided descriptive insight on functions and possible effects. As well, eight primary emotions (anger, anxiety, shame, guilt, hope, relief, happiness, and pride) were discussed in detail and are strikingly similar to the seven emotions identified by Vallerand's (1983) review of emotion in sport (happiness, surprise, fear, anger, sadness, disgust/contempt, and interest). Effects of these emotions have been observed in Olympic environments (Botterill, 1996), and the implications regarding the relevant emotional preparation and emotional management strategies for teams and individuals will be discussed in detail later in the chapter.

Hanin's (2000) work helped us recognize that everyone has an individual zone of optimal functioning (IZOF). Furthermore, individual perception plays a big role regarding the effects of emotions. Team strategies can play a tremendous role in preparing for and managing emotions, but individual differences regarding emotional effects need to be respected. Hanin recommends that performers "keep book" on themselves to uncover which positive and negative emotions are functional and which are dysfunctional in specific circumstances. Hackfort (1995) has also recommended that a careful functional analysis be required in order to avoid inappropriate assumptions about individual perceptions regarding affect. As he points out, "There are no good or bad, positive or negative emotions per se" (p. 28).

There is an immense interest in emotional intelligence (Goleman, 1998) in the worlds of business and education. Sosik and Megerian (1999) point to an important relationship between emotional intelligence and effective leadership. There is probably little doubt in sport and beyond that those able to harness and manage their emotions under pressure are going to be perceived as the most effective leaders. It would appear that the most successful teams must possess both quality leadership and emotional intelligence.

Recent in-depth interview studies of top performers (Brown, 2001; Newburg, 1998) have explored the kind of "perspective" that leads to inner peace, confidence, and emotional mastery. Initial data suggest that early experiences play an important role, but that self-awareness and a more rational perspective can be pursued and accomplished at any stage of life. Sadly, Kübler-Ross and Kessler (2000) point out that many of us do not appreciate the key lessons of life until we face death.

Emotions are most certainly a qualitative topic. As Tenenbaum (1995) suggests, the challenges of the new millennium are likely to require progressive research and application methodologies. Feelings are powerfully related to health and performance in sport, and most likely it will take an authentic, team effort to master this topic.

Understanding Emotions

Defining emotions has always proven troublesome, and such a task is no easier today (Martin, 1996; Vallerand & Blanchard, 2000). Although a number of definitions and positions exist, a simple, straightforward discussion is really what is required when discussing this phenomenon with those who participate in sport.

Glasser (1984) identified the four components of total behavior as physiology, feeling, thinking, and doing. All of these components interact and influence one another. For example, managing one's physiology can have an impact on athletes' respective feeling, which can then influence their thinking and possibly how they will eventually perform (doing). Emotion can be viewed as related to all of these components, as they all appear to have dynamic two-way relationships. The spontaneous dimension of emotions, however, makes them much more difficult to manage.

Emotion is experienced as a physiological and psychological reaction to an event, which can either exist in reality or be a product of someone's thinking about a past, present, or upcoming situation. The feeling that an athlete may experience before the start of a competition ("butterflies"), the frustration that is experienced after a loss, and the anger that one may feel after finding oneself on the receiving end of an aggressive play are all common examples of emotional situations in sport that evoke these internal, physiological, and psychological sensations.

Once the event and the corresponding emotions have occurred, we then express ourselves consistently with our prior learning of how to interpret and then label the emotions. For example, athletes can label high levels of activation as either excitement or nervousness, depending on their past experiences and how those experiences were reinforced.

Emotional Preparation

Perhaps the best way to appreciate emotions and their importance to effective preparation is to ask how they differ from mental preparation. In team sports it is often the difference between what can be referred to as "blue-collar" preparation and "white-collar" preparation. Both involve mental rehearsal, but white-collar preparation often assumes that everything will go right. As a result, many of the emotions and feelings that might occur in a competition are not "triggered."

If the full range of possible emotional feelings are triggered and strong effective responses, rehearsed, a form of "emotional inoculation" and readiness is accomplished. Athletes and teams need to anticipate situations and challenges that will trigger at least the seven basic categories of emotions that Vallerand (1984) outlined. This should be done systematically, and each feeling "triggered" should be followed by the rehearsal of a "quality" physical, mental, and emotional response.

This exercise should be completed well ahead of the competition so that the athlete (and the team) feel totally ready for the challenges of competition during the countdown hours. Emotional preparation can be included with mental rehearsal of the "game plan" early on game day, with more thorough contingency planning occurring the night before.

Most athletes are disciplined enough to do their mental and physical preparation, but when their preparation is inadequate or ineffective, it is usually because their emotional preparation was neglected (Botterill, 1996). On the other hand, it is not "natural" to want to scare oneself and trigger the full range of emotions for every competition—especially if the athlete is tired or complacent from schedule demands. Several of the emotions that top competitors need to be ready for are negative, and it takes enormous professional discipline to prepare for the full range of emotions on every occasion.

Important Emotions to Be Ready For

Surprise is probably the first emotion for which to be ready. Top performers and teams expect their opponent's best and most annoying performance. They expect surprising and annoying circumstances and demands, and they rehearse effective responses ahead of time. It is also important to be ready for positive as well as negative surprise. Many teams have not been ready for a surprisingly effective start and have gone on to be vulnerable as a result of a drop in focus and work ethic.

Surprise in the score, the opponents, teammates, the officiating, the crowds, the conditions, timing delays, and last-minute changes are examples of situations to be ready for. Emotional readiness for surprise is often the key to success in the dramatic world of sport.

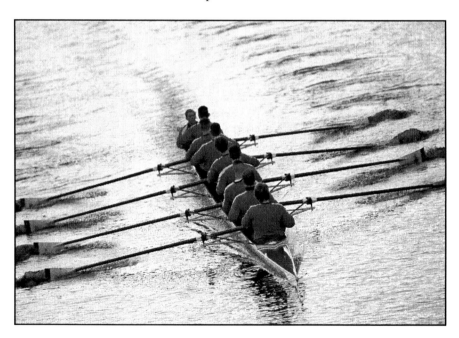

Good athletes must be able to adapt to the unique conditions of each event.

Negative surprise is often combined with feelings of fear, anger, and sometimes guilt or embarrassment. It is important to have triggered all of these emotions ahead of time and to have rehearsed effective responses for each. Fear of failure can initially be functional, but it is important to have rehearsed "pursuing success" rather than trying to "avoid failure" in response to this feeling. Pat Riley of the NBA's Miami Heat proclaimed that the difference between their teams when they play "to win" versus "not to lose" is like night and day (Riley, 1993). It is important to anticipate situations where one may be prone to "fear of failure" and to rehearse effective coping responses.

Anger can be functional if it helps athletes fight for what they are entitled to, but many games have been lost when anger has produced a loss of focus, lack of discipline, and selfishness. Again, it is important to trigger the potential feelings from possible anger-producing possibilities ahead of time and rehearse energetic but disciplined and focused responses.

Guilt and embarrassment can also contribute to a loss of focus, as one becomes self-conscious and sometimes distracted by related feelings of shame and anger. It is important to anticipate situations where opponents or one's own performance might make an athlete feel guilty and embarrassed and to rehearse quality responses. These situations should simply be a trigger to work hard for one's teammates (and for oneself) and to focus even better on the task at hand.

Low-Energy Emotion

One emotion that an athlete cannot afford to dwell on for very long in a competition is sadness. On the other hand, momentary disappointment, compassion for an injured teammate, and off-field tragedies are realities of life that are bound to trigger this emotion. It is important not to deny sadness, because it is an important part of grieving—which eventually leads to feelings of gratitude and optimism as we try to get over events that have happened to us.

However, because sadness is low energy and usually involves feeling sorry for oneself or others, it is in most cases a problem sentiment in high-performance sport. Nevertheless, performers can actually be "inspired" in the face of disappointment or tragedy. Promising oneself that one can delay grieving until later can sometimes help maintain focus and energy, but rehearsing quality responses to disappointment ahead of time is often the key to being able to perform when it is important. This process was extremely important for the Canadian Women's National Volleyball Team in the fall of 1998.

While the team was in preparation for an international volleyball tournament being held at home in Canada, the fiancé of one of the players succumbed to cancer. All who were involved with the team felt this sudden and tragic event, and his youth (he was 30 years of age when he passed away) made the event difficult to accept and process. The tournament was not going to be delayed or cancelled, and it was up to the players and coaching staff to accept their own feelings and to make a decision to continue grieving only after the tournament was over. By delaying the experiencing of profound sadness until after the competition, the team was able to maintain an effective energy "reserve" that made possible an appearance in the final. The team was able to perform through demanding competitive circumstances, including a comeback win from being down two games to none against the Dominican Republic.

To effectively delay the process of remorse and sadness, a "remember the highlights" theme was adopted. Players were encouraged to initially accept their natural emotional responses and then to focus their energies on all of the great things that the player's fiancé had brought to their team and to the community. This helped to keep emotions positive until the tournament was over. At the end of the tournament, the fatigue and level of emotion experienced by the team were overwhelming.

Throughout the experience, guilt needed to be addressed and managed so that the players could give themselves permission to play despite having experienced such a great loss. Although not as common as other emotions in sport, sadness must also be appreciated and prepared for so that effective coping strategies and responses can be nurtured and developed.

Orlick (1998) proposed a number of useful steps to follow to aid in facilitating effective transitions from setbacks and emotional challenges. They include
- Expect a down time or period of adaptation—it is normal.
- Allow time for rest and relaxation.
- Take the time to be caressed, refreshed, and rejuvenated by nature, loved ones, and simple joys.
- Stay active but slow things down.
- Explain to loved ones that you may need some time alone, time with nature, or support from others to resurface.
- Expect to return to a more positive state of mind and, with time, to be ready to embrace new opportunities and face whatever challenges lie ahead.
- Follow your heart.

Not all emotions are negative. It is also important to be ready for excessive positive emotions. Excessive happiness and interest in novel circumstances can affect focus as a result of temporary complacency or distraction. If these feelings have been triggered ahead of time and a quality response rehearsed, the situations involved become reminders to focus and finish. When one is properly emotionally prepared, these emotions will dominate, thus resulting in performers who are simply enjoying the challenge of the game.

There are other emotions like jealousy and resentment that perhaps one should also be ready for, but most of the other emotions are derivatives or combinations of the seven basic emotions discussed. If the players have triggered the basic emotions as part of their preparation and rehearsed effective responses, they are then likely to be ready and able to handle the full range of emotions that are possible in sport.

Emotional Preparation and Teams

In team sport, it is the responsibility of the players to teammates and to themselves to be vigilant and thorough regarding the emotional preparation that becomes critical for effective feelings of "team" readiness. Sometimes all it takes is one athlete who is not ready for the feelings generated in a game to cost a victory. Collective emotional readiness, on the other hand, is extremely powerful, and teammates and opponents often feel the deep "feelings" of readiness. Depth of readiness and belief is often the difference in close match-ups. Collective and individual emotional preparation plays a critical role in this difference.

Riley (1993) advanced an appreciation of the emotional stages involved in the overall emotional preparation of a team. When groups "form," tremendous turmoil results until we are comfortable with our role on the team. Of utmost importance is Riley's "disease of me" that results when personal needs compete or interfere with team needs. This phenomenon can be found on both successful and unsuccessful teams alike. An effective strategy for overcoming the "disease of me" is the development of a "core covenant."

A core covenant results when one trusts that whatever is good for the team is also good for oneself. It is, in a sense, a team's mission statement. The most important values that the players and coaches should work towards involve cooperation, love, hard work, and total concentration on the "good of the team." The "norming" properties of a core covenant occur once everyone on the team realizes he or she is needed and appreciated. This can help make the emotions that may be experienced in demanding situations manageable. Athletes engage in more supportive communication if challenged and realize that their teammate "cares" about the team, which helps them to accept in a constructive manner the criticism from a teammate or coach.

In completing "emotional inoculation," players should anticipate situations and contrasting conditions that might trigger various emotional responses. These feelings need to be triggered for every game and effective responses rehearsed to ensure a broad effective concentration zone by everyone who is on the team.

Emotional preparation is easy to neglect—sometimes it seems like human nature to do so. It is, however, a big part of being and becoming "exceptional." It needs to be taught so that many more individuals and teams are able to come closer to their potential.

Emotional Management

Another important component of emotion and performance involves "emotional management." There are three important aspects of "fitness" to work on and maintain for optimal sport performances. Each aspect of fitness involves "capacities" and a "state." Physical fitness, for example, needs to be developed and maintained through a balance of stress and rest so that key physical capacities are fostered and maintained without draining physical, mental, or emotional reserves due to overtraining. Emphasis shifts from quantity to quality training; appropriate hydration, nutrition, and rest patterns are extremely beneficial in helping optimize one's physical, mental, and emotional state.

Mental Fitness

Good fitness management, however, dictates that there is enough quality training and "work" for therapeutic effects, confidence, and concentration. Mental fitness is also a set of capacities and a state. It is important to work on and maintain one's mental skills. Imagery, relaxation, energizing, "parking" distractions, focusing, relationship management, and time management can all play critical roles as one refines them as part of precompetition routines (see chapter 4), competition focus plans, refocusing strategies (see chapter 9 for information on concentration techniques), and postperformance evaluations.

Once again, though, it is important to ensure that one does not allow oneself to become overloaded with too many cognitive or mental demands throughout a competitive season or during long periods of training. The resulting overload, stress, and distraction can mask an athlete's mental skills the same way physical overload or poor nutrition can mask his or her physical capacities. The result, of course, can be emotional, mental, and physical staleness.

Being clear-minded should be an important objective going into the competition. This will help to avoid falling into the human tendency to start "over-analysing." It has been suggested that "nothing never happens" — in the absence of a constructive focus we sometimes start "overthinking" or "overperceiving."

One should be confident in one's mental skills going into a competition. Responses to stress and boredom should automatically be constructive, and time and relationship skills should be crisp and effective. Creative simulations, quality training sessions, and lead-up competitions can help ensure that the attentional and competitive skills will be close to their potential.

Emotional Readiness and Fitness

Simulations also play a critical role in developing one's emotional fitness. By simulating and rehearsing responses to some of the most demanding, distracting or emotionally disturbing possibilities, we can test our emotional skills, capacities, and responses. Simulations allow us to practice our desired performance responses and coping strategies in circumstances that are as authentic as we can make them before we actually have to perform in the real situation (Orlick, 2001). It may not always be "fun" as we prepare for the full spectrum of emotional possibilities, but with practice, the development of an inner confidence in our capacities to maintain our focus and to respond effectively will be facilitated.

With preparation, we become "mentally tough" and learn to accept, harness, and respond to the full spectrum of emotions. We can begin to realize that all emotions are functional and "manage" them much better. We become emotionally resilient knowing we can call on a wide range of emotions for energy and appropriate feelings.

Like the other two areas of fitness, it is critical that one not allow oneself to become emotionally drained prior to or during a competition. Once again, an athlete's emotional skills and capacities can be eroded if the emotional state is allowed to deteriorate. As well, it is important to remember that emotional recovery involves not only resting but also doing stimulating things that we enjoy.

Postperformance Evaluations (Emotional Debriefing)

Another very important emotional management technique has to do with our ability to evaluate all of our performances objectively. Too often in sport, we evaluate only our competitive performance opportunities, often neglecting the importance of processing our emotions on a daily basis. This is necessary if we are to prevent episodes of chronic stress, which is so often associated with burnout in athletes and coaches (Smith, 1986). Through daily debriefing routines, frustrating situations that occur during training can be resolved, instances of miscommunication can be clarified, and goals for the next practice can be established. Teams (and individuals) should be encouraged to ask themselves two important questions:

What went well today?

What can we improve upon tomorrow?

The result is a team that has a balanced perception of all performance opportunities, regardless of the outcome of the training session or competition.

Finally, debriefing can provide important daily communication opportunities between teammates in less stress-evoking situations. This can help coaches and athletes share their thoughts on the team's performance and level of goal achievement in a more rational but assertive manner. It can improve a team's ability to "norm" in a continuous way throughout a season and can help to avoid relationship "peaks" and "valleys" throughout a season.

Emotional exhaustion is probably the key component in burnout, overtraining, etc. It is amazing what human beings can do physically and mentally, but it is usually emotional exhaustion that buries them. Therefore, it is critical to make "emotional management" an important part of fitness and overall training and competition preparation strategy.

There have been stories of phenomenal emotional resilience in sport: Witness Canadian synchronized swimmer Sylvie Frechette's performance at the 1992 Olympics after her fiancé's suicide—and her classy response after initially losing the gold medal on a judging system error (TSN.ca/olympics/history/1992.asp; 1992). There are phenomenal stories that demonstrate that we can sometimes draw on "emotional reserves" that we do not even know we have.

On the other hand, someone going into a major competition striving for a "personal best" in a very emotional environment would be best advised to try to be sure his or her emotional reserves are not depleted. If possible, relationships with loved ones, school or career demands, health risks, opponent hostilities, financial pressures, community or environmental concerns, and media pressures should be managed in a way to minimize emotional drain prior to and during the competition.

Managing Our Emotional Health

Another important part of emotional management involves periodic checks of one's perspective. It is important to be on a "mission" to accomplish a personal best, but in light of all the "hype," aura, and mystique of elite sport, it is critical to maintain a rational perspective.

Checking to ensure irrational beliefs or perceptions do not develop can prevent a lot of potential emotional turmoil and pressure. It is easy to exaggerate the perceived importance of competitions to the point where we start feeling "our self-worth and life are on the line." Championships are an exciting opportunity, but we should never feel they determine our worth as human beings. That is determined in so many other ways. Witness Norwegian speed skater, Johan Olaf Koss, and his "life beyond sport"—raising support for hospitals and charities and pursuing meaningful career opportunities.

Similarly, American speed skater Dan Janssen's accomplishments as an Olympian pale in comparison to the relationships with his family, including the loss of his sister to cancer and the love and support of his family through this heartbreak in the pursuit of excellence.

Feelings of patriotism and responsibility to others can lead to thinking that one "must perform for others." Narrowing this perception and pressure to wanting to perform for oneself and teammates is much more rational and emotionally less stressful.

The high standards and ideals of sport can also lead to feelings that "I must be perfect." Perfection by definition and reality is impossible, so it is important to rationally remind oneself that sport is about "the pursuit of excellence." Striving for situational, personal, and team excellence is what it is all about, and if mistakes, setbacks, or challenges occur in a competition or throughout a season it is important to be ready to enjoy the challenge of responding optimally.

Finally, with the stakes so high, we can begin to expect that "things will and must be fair." However, scrutiny reveals countless competitive situations that do not appear personally or professionally fair. The judging mishap in Sylvie Frechette's 1992 Olympic case in synchronized swimming or Mary Decker's fall due to crowding in the 1984 Olympics middle distance athletics event are examples in which the world just does not seem fair.

It is important, then, to be prepared for the possibility that one may not always have a level playing field and be prepared to respond to adversity if it should present itself. An expectation that everything will always be fair can lead to considerable emotional frustration and fluctuation. On the other hand, someone who has developed a "no excuses" outlook and has prepared to handle the many challenges and emotions of competition is more likely to accomplish a "personal best."

Cliff Wurtak, an elite ringette coach preparing for the Canada Winter Games, suggested his athletes adopt a simple outlook in preparing for and participating in the games: "Never have to say I wish I would have."

This sentiment clearly suggests that it is important to do everything possible to physically, mentally, and emotionally prepare oneself for competition. It also suggests that one should be ready to be assertive, to "play with license," and to make the most of the opportunities presented. Finally, this outlook suggests that one should be ready to fully experience and respond to the emotions and challenges of training and competition.

Macro Time Management

In order to regularly and efficiently concentrate and focus, we need to look after ourselves in a variety of ways. If we manage well only those moments of training, development, and competition, our ability to do so in the future will eventually deteriorate (Botterill & Patrick, 1996). Physical and mental health as well as overall life focus has to be monitored in order to repeatedly and consistently manage emotions effectively in as many situations as possible.

Blocks of time to rest, relax, reenergize, and pursue other interests and relationships can be critical to a performer's long-term ability to manage his or her emotion and performance demands effectively. As human beings, we all have a need for a reasonable balance in our activities and pursuits. Those pursuing excellence in a given field can often focus tremendous energy and effort in particular pursuits over significant periods of time. However, the ability to effectively do so over extended periods can deteriorate if basic human needs and balance are neglected. Due to the intensity and demands of training and development programs in sport, athletes need to be encouraged to maintain some balance (other interests) and long-term focus in their lives.

Too often, we neglect the role of our "self." We often assume that spending time in relationships with friends or significant others is helping us get away from the demands of sport, but what we really must monitor is that we have enough time alone to reflect, and more important, relax.

Athletes or coaches should actively manage (or co-manage) different aspects of their technical, tactical, physical, mental, and emotional preparation and development in order to produce transferable lifetime skills and knowledge. Although physical skills may deteriorate with age, the mental and emotional skills necessary to be a good "time and relationship manager" can be developed in any situation and transferred to a wide variety of professions, lifetime activities, and challenging situations. If performers recognize and pursue their potential in other interests and relationships, they will end up with a broader identity, focus, and capability. This makes them less prone to dramatic shifts in feelings of worthlessness and low self-confidence. This "broader" focus also helps performers to stay rational and to concentrate when necessary, because they are more likely to keep things in perspective and maintain feelings of balance and control.

Macro time management requires us to consider all the roles we play and to seek a balance among these roles over time. It is not necessary (or possible) to achieve complete horizontal balance in our roles every week or month. We must expect, for example, to spend more time in sport when we are pursuing it as a career, or when training towards an ultimate goal of a medal performance at a World Championship or Olympic Games. The key is to have vertical or longitudinal balance in life. This can be achieved by effective long-term planning, thus allowing performers to maintain perspective as they experience their busy lives. Maintaining "threads" of meaningful activity related to one's identity beyond sport is important. For example, student-athletes with career aspirations may take only one course (by correspondence) the year of the Olympics. Similarly, hard-working coaches may need to plan quality time with their families (both off season and in season) in order to maintain balance and perspective.

Summary

The goal of most performers is to walk away knowing they gave it their best shot and remain thrilled about the opportunity to test themselves in one of the most prestigious and emotional environments in the world…SPORT! We must accept that we can never totally control our emotions—that is part of the challenge of being "human." With emotional preparation, practice, and management, we can often come much closer to our performance potential and enjoy the rewards of knowing that we did everything possible to achieve our goals. We can learn to accept our feelings and use their energy or simply let them go and look ahead towards the possibilities that the next opportunity will hold in store for us.

References

Botterill, C. (1996). Emotional preparation in the Olympic games. *Coaches Report, 3,* 26-30.

Botterill, C., & Patrick, T. (1996). *Human potential: Perspective, passion, & preparation.* Winnipeg: Lifeskills.

Brown, M. (2001). *The process of perspective.* Unpublished doctoral dissertation, University of Calgary, Calgary, Alberta, Canada.

Crocker, P. R. E., Alderman, R. B., & Smith, M. R. (1988). Cognitive-affective stress management training with high performance youth volleyball players: Effects on affect, cognition, and performance. *Journal of Sport & Exercise Psychology, 10,* 448-460.

Glasser, W. (1984). *Control theory.* New York: Harper and Row.

Goleman, D. (1995). *Emotional intelligence.* New York: Bantam Books.

Goleman, D. (1998). *Working with emotional intelligence.* New York: Bantam Books.

Hackfort, D. (1995). Emotion in sports: A functional analysis out of the action theory perspective. In F. H. Fu & M. L. Ng (Eds.), *Sport psychology: Perspectives and practices toward the 21st century* (pp. 27-34). Hong Kong: Glory Printing & Productions.

Hanin, Y. (2000). Individual zones of optimal functioning (IZOF) model: Emotion-performance relationships in sport. In Y. Hanin (Ed.), *Emotions in sport* (pp. 65-89). Champaign, IL: Human Kinetics.

Hanin, Y., & Syrja, P. (1995). Performance affect in junior ice hockey players: An application of the individual zones of optimal functioning model. *The Sport Psychologist, 9,* 169-187.

Hassmen, P., & Blomstrand, E. (1995). Mood state relationships and soccer team performance. *The Sport Psychologist, 9,* 297-308.

Kübler-Ross, E., & Kessler, D. (2000). *Life lessons.* New York: Scribner.

Lazarus, R. S. (2000). How emotions influence performance in competitive sports. *The Sport Psychologist, 14,* 229-252.

Martin, G. L. (1996). *Sport psychology consulting: Practical guidelines from behavior analysis.* Manitoba: University of Manitoba.

Newburg, D. S. (1998). *Resonance - A life by design: Developing your dream and mastering your fear.* Unpublished manuscript.

Orlick, T. (1998). *Embracing your potential.* Champaign, IL: Human Kinetics.

Orlick, T. (2001). *In pursuit of excellence* (2nd ed.). Champaign, IL: Leisure Press.

Prapavessis, H., & Grove, J. R. (1991). Precompetitive emotions and shooting per-formance: The mental health and zone of optimal function models. *The Sport Psychologist, 5,* 223-234.

Riley, P. (1993). *The winner within: A life plan for team players.* New York, NY: G. P. Putnam.

Smith, R. E. (1986). Toward a cognitive-affective model of athletic burnout. *Journal of Sport Psychology, 8,* 36-50.

Sosik, J., & Megerian, L. (1999). Understanding leader emotional intelligence and performance: The role of self-other agreement on transformational leadership perceptions. *Group & Organization Management, 24,* 367-391.

Tenenbaum, G. (1995). Methodological considerations in sport psychology: Current status and future directions. In F. H. Fu & M. L. Ng (Eds.), *Sport psy-chology: Perspectives and practices toward the 21st century* (pp. 3-20). Hong Kong: Glory Printing & Productions.

Terry, P. (1995). The efficacy of mood state profiling with elite performers: A review and synthesis. *The Sport Psychologist, 9,* 309-324.

TSN.ca/olympics/history/1992.asp; 1992. "1992 Olympic Games XXV" TSN.ca, Barcelona, Spain, August. Available on-line.

Vallerand, R. J. (1983). On emotion in sport: Theoretical and social psychological perspectives. *Journal of Sport Psychology, 5,* 197-215.

Vallerand, R. J., & Blanchard, C. M. (2000). The study of emotion in sport and exercise: Historical, definitional, and conceptual perspectives. In Y. Hanin (Ed.), *Emotions in sport* (pp. 3-37). Champaign, IL: Human Kinetics.

CHAPTER 7

Gender Differences When Working With Men's and Women's Teams

Gloria Balague

Abstract

The role of a sport psychologist when consulting, traveling, and generally working with individual athletes is often complex and ill defined (Balague, Taylor, LeScanff, & Botterill, 1997). Each athlete is unique and therefore requires special treatment. Even more complex, though, is the role of the sport psychologist when working with team sports because subtle interpersonal issues combine with individual factors to influence the performance of the whole group. It is the primary purpose of this chapter to thoroughly discuss some of these interpersonal issues and individual factors that frequently occur on athletic teams, according to gender. Men's and women's athletic teams may be faced with similar problems, but how they usually deal with them is vastly different. So, a secondary purpose of this chapter is to suggest some interventions that are effective in remedying these issues and problems—again according to gender.

The influence of gender in behavior and performance in sport has not been widely researched. Tuffy (1996) summarized gender differences in sport after conducting an extensive review of the literature. She noted differences in reporting of anxiety (higher for females), small differences in self-confidence (higher for males in the physical domain), no differences in causal attribution, and some differences in achievement motivation and leadership style—but not necessarily with elite-level athletes. Differences in aggression and communication have been demonstrated empirically but not in the sport domain.

In her research, Tuffy (1996) interviewed 14 college coaches, who successfully coached both male and female athletes, about their perception of the differences between male and female athletes. Overall, the coaches acknowledged that female and male athletes are more similar than different, but also that there were some ways in which female and male athletes differed that affected the coach-athlete interaction. Coaches perceived female athletes as being more emotional and expressing emotions differently and also as having a higher need for social validation. Coaches also felt that they tended to be more direct in their communication with male athletes; they also perceived males as having a lesser need for a strong relationship with their coach, whereas females wanted and needed more from their coaches than the "technical" aspects of coaching. Tuffy's research opens a number of interesting issues for follow-up, including the assessment of how sport psychologists view male and female athletes. The following chapter is based mainly on my observations of these issues.

Issues in Working With Teams

Communication

Overall, one of the most noticeable problems I have observed when working with women's teams has been the issue of communication difficulties and their impact on the team. In my experience, women athletes have difficulty giving each other positive and helpful feedback. They seem to fear offending a teammate and will not give technical corrections or feedback, such as "toss that ball more to the right" or "follow me closely when the defender moves back." Women also tend to take strong offense when receiving such feedback from a teammate; this, in turn, affects their intensity and ability to bounce back from mistakes.

One of the national teams I have worked with had a great opportunity to reflect on this issue after they had a chance to practice with some of the men's team members, and the women's team decided to make some changes in that area. The players observed how the men provided concrete feedback and even yelled directions during play, without having any personal implications. The result was an increase in the level and intensity of the play of the women's team members and also an increased awareness of how they would have reacted differently if that same information had come from a female teammate.

Another type of miscommunication, seen in both male and female teams but more prevalent in women's teams, has to do with nonverbal communication. Athletes often become frustrated with their own performance, and some translate this into specific body and facial gestures (i.e., rolling their eyes, throwing the equipment, kicking the ground). Women athletes seem to have a harder time reading these behaviors of teammates as unrelated to themselves.

That is, when another player, particularly one with whom they have had some negative interactions in the games or practices, makes a face, thus showing disgust or rolling her eyes, many women players feel that this player is mad or upset at them in a much greater proportion than do the men players. Other behaviors manifested later on compound the problem because these players never check out their assumption that the teammate is actually mad at them. Consequently, they act hurt in return, therefore creating an interpersonal conflict because of the misperceptions.

Finally, another communication problem more prevalent among women is that of indirect communication and rumors. Women athletes appear to display rivalry with a teammate by talking about that teammate to others and creating and divulging rumors, which result in the formation of "negative cliques" that cause dissension in the team. Men tend to display rivalry more directly on the field or in the locker room. Occasionally, this takes the form of verbal "ribbing" and joking. Men's rivalry with a teammate who shares the same position is sometimes manifested as "head games"; that is, making comments to increase the level of pressure felt by the other player or reminding him of something that is a problem. Men will say things such as "do not think about failing" to a player who fears failure.

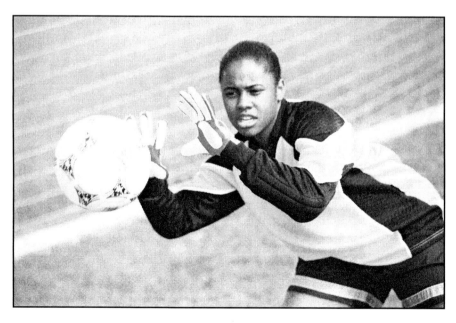

When dealing with team disputes, remember that miscommunication takes different forms among women than it does with men.

Interventions for communication. With women's teams I have found basic communication training and open discussions on any subject to be highly effective. It is also helpful to encourage that the usage of "I" statements be descriptive rather than judgmental and that the players practice active listening to the message (Dinkmeyer & Losoney, 1980; McKay, Davis, & Fanning, 1983). To break the habit of talking about other players, a team discussion and a team agreement to change that behavior, including accepting responsibility for the fact that listening to gossip about another player perpetuates the problem, are essential tools. These team discussions must have a concrete outcome and specific follow-up, or the resolutions are very short-lived. For some of the men's teams, I have found it useful to encourage more communication and reinforce positive feedback. Giving opportunities to list specific things that each member of the team contributes to the group performance allows for concrete positive information for each player. Often, individual work with the player who is the target of someone else's undermining comments is a most helpful intervention.

Past History of Success and Failure

The past history of success and failure in competition with certain opponents is something that affects both men's and women's teams, but I have observed a difference in how it is manifested according to gender. Women's teams appear much more vulnerable to the attitude of the team leaders. Veteran players, with a longer history against certain opponents, seem to carry much more weight on women's teams. If the veteran players have a negative history against certain teams and play in a more timid, defensive manner, then younger players on women's teams appear reluctant to step over the veteran leaders, even though the younger players themselves may not be particularly intimidated by the opposing team. In men's teams, the team may be intimidated by an opponent, but the reaction does not appear to be so clearly related to the behaviors of the veteran players.

Interventions for success and failure. I have found this to be one of the most complex issues in team sports. The chemistry of the team is delicate and can rapidly change. (The reader can find a discussion on some aspects of the chemistry of a team in chapter 5.)

For the women's teams, I believe that it is important not to create a rift between the "young" and the "veteran" players; thus the intervention needed is to ensure that there is no finger-pointing from one group to the other. The use of video has proven helpful, as players are asked to individually view a film of the game or competition and indicate specific things each one would do differently at critical moments (emphasizing decision making). A second viewing of the video allows for mixed groups of players (veteran, younger, different positions) to review it and make specific suggestions according to positions (forwards, guards, etc.), thus acknowledging and using the information already provided by the individual player's reviews. For men's teams, team discussions of both the individual players' game plans as well as an overall team plan appear to be enough.

Selection Issues

Being a starter versus being a nonstarter is a chronic source of frustration for many team players. Again I have found differences in how men and women react to this situation. A reminder here is that several of the women's teams I have worked with were national teams, composed of players who were all "stars" of their original clubs or teams; this may have significantly colored my perceptions by attributing more importance to gender when it is perhaps just a team composition issue. Having stated the previous disclaimer, I had the overall impression that women have stronger emotional reactions to not being selected as starters than do men. Women also often take the selection personally, as if the coach means to ridicule them; thus they react with lowered motivation and statements such as "what is the point" or "I do not want to play for this coach." If the emotional reaction is strong, the behavioral response is also frequently counterproductive. The players who feel "wronged" by not starting tend to sulk and distance themselves as much as possible from the coach. They will physically sit at the farthest end of the bench, avoid eye contact, etc., and thus minimize their chances of being noticed by the coach or selected to play sooner. Men athletes, on the other hand, are also often mad at not being selected, but this fact does not seem to affect their motivation in the same way. On the contrary, they want to show the coach that they are better players and often approach him to find out what they need to do to improve in order to regain their starting status.

    Interventions for selection issues. With women's teams, the most effective intervention is through the coach. If the coach is willing to publicly acknowledge that there are several players that have been considered as starters and provide some overall comments describing the reasoning underlying the specific choices, such as "Today we need more speed, so I will go with X" or just acknowledge the hard work or good efforts of some of the other players who were not chosen, the problems will be minimal. On some occasions, though, coaches will not be willing to make these statements because they feel that these are pure coaching decisions that they should not have to justify. In those cases, it may become necessary to work with the nonstarting athlete and make her aware that her negative reactions will only hurt her and her chances to increase playing time in the future. Cognitive restructuring, working on their interpretations of the "meaning" they attribute to the coach's decisions, and making behavioral assignments to actually increase eye contact and availability to the coach are also quite successful interventions. For men's teams, helping athletes prepare for their individual meeting with the coach, if they want to discuss how to increase their chances of starting, is the intervention that is most effective.

Personal Life Issues

Long training camps and road trips make personal life issues very salient to the morale of team sports. The main difference I have observed in how various teams handle this issue has more to do with age and experience than with gender. Younger players miss home, friends, and their familiar environments. In many cases, even the physical environment is a key piece in their adaptation. Some players miss the mountains or the open air or the city life, depending on what their frame of reference has been. Older players, often with established relationships, tend to miss their partners and home life, as well as the intellectual stimulation provided by their professional colleagues or peers. One specific issue that is developing as more women have access to professional careers in sport is the issue of the psychological adaptation of those women athletes who have children. This is not to imply that male athletes who are fathers do not miss their children, but I have had a chance to interview numerous female athletes who have children, and the issues of guilt over their absence, self-labeling as selfish for pursuing an athletic endeavor, and sadness over the separation were pervasive and often interfered with performance (Vernacchia, Balague, Yambor, & Shaw, 1995). Numerous individual athletes have found a way to combine athletics and motherhood, by sometimes bringing the children along with a caretaker or arranging for short visits. In the case of team sports, the flexibility over living quarters and travel schedules is not as great, and satisfactory solutions may not be readily available.

Relationship/Sexuality Issues

Relationships and sexuality issues are a major source of emotional turmoil for people in general, and particularly for young adults. When some of the athletes on a team experience intense emotional reactions, it can result in problems in team cohesion, morale, and performance. When the conflict is between two or more players or when it involves the coach and some players, the consequences are likely to be very disruptive for the whole team. Comparing men's and women's teams, I have found a phenomenon that has great relevance to team dynamics but is not often discussed in the sport psychology literature. Some women's teams have a number of homosexual players, and a percentage of coaches are also homosexual. In some cases, the sport environment is the first place where they have felt the freedom to discuss their sexual orientation and/or where they have made friends who share the same sexual orientation. Sometimes this results in a number of intense, closed relationships that change the nature of the group. In some cases these relationships involve younger players experiment-ing with sexual identity issues. By default then, these are unstable relationships that are likely to change rapidly. The breakup of such liaisons is also likely to coin-cide with moments of maximum stress, usually around the most important tour-naments and/or games. All of this means that months of collective work by the whole team can be neutralized by a relationship conflict. In teams where there is a wide range of age and experience, another disruptive scenario I have observed is that of a dominant partner controlling a more submissive one. Depending on how sexual orientation is handled by the team, some of the players may feel unwelcome because of their sexual orientation. The result is divisiveness within the team and decrements in performance, not to mention unhappiness and lack of personal growth. In her insightful book *Coming on Strong*, Cahn (1994) described the mixed messages received by lesbian athletes in sport:

> ...From at least the 1940s on, sport provided space for lesbians to gather and build shared culture. Lesbians could not publicly claim their identity without risking expulsion, ostracism, and loss of athletic activities and social networks that had become crucial to their sense of well being.... Concealment and secrecy provid-ed a degree of protection and flexibility. But, crucially, this strat-egy also kept lesbianism underground; ...the lesbian culture of sport formed an "open secret" in American society, operating on —but not challenging—the fine line between public knowledge and practiced ignorance. (pp. 205)

Homosexual relationships within the team are no more disruptive than heterosexual relationships in the workplace (Griffin, 1998). It is really not about the sexual relationship itself, but about the existence of a closed unit within the team, and the same level of disruption would be caused by two heterosexual players involved with the same partner and experiencing an intense conflict because of it. The team should address these relationship issues because eventually they will affect the whole team. As a sport psychologist, this is the part I found most puzzling: People were very unwilling to address these issues. Traditionally, sport psychology has also failed to discuss this issue in this context. Specific issues and psychological pressures faced by lesbian or gay athletes have been addressed by a minority of researchers (Krane, 1996; Messner, 1992), but researchers have not considered the group dynamics and performance effects. In men's teams I have witnessed on occasion very closed subgroups that were interfering with the team dynamics. I am sure that there are gay athletes who may form a relationship with a teammate, but the frequency of this phenomenon is definitely lower and the impact on the team is often much less because male homosexual athletes face great pressure to hide such information from everyone else, thus making it unlikely that they will form a very visible subgroup.

Another primary issue that can greatly affect team cohesion and morale, as well as the psychological well-being of the athletes, is that of intimate relationships between coaches and athletes. I have witnessed this happening in a variety of combinations—male coaches with female athletes, female coaches with female athletes, male coaches with male athletes—and it can occur with female coaches and male athletes. Two major issues are of concern here.

The first one has to do with the uneven power in the relationship. The coach has power over the athlete, even if the athlete is of legal age. The coach can make decisions that affect the future of the athlete in terms of selection, playing time, etc. The coach is often admired and respected because of the position he or she holds, independent of the person the coach is. All of this means that the athlete cannot really make a choice of whether he or she wants the relationship. This situation is, of course, wrong and can have long-lasting, negative consequences for the athlete as well as the team.

The second aspect is that of the disruption in team dynamics when the coach and one of the players form a separate unit or when athletes feel that the coach's technical decisions are heavily determined by his or her relationship with one player. The team's communication patterns and general atmosphere are interrupted, and the results are, among other things, demoralization of the team, lack of trust in the coach, and anger and resentment at the coach and the player involved.

Interventions for sexuality issues. One of the main interventions I have used for this issue is that of opening up the topic for discussion. There never should be an issue that affects everyone that is officially kept covered up. I have found that helping the team discuss what kind of team they want to be and how important athletic performance is to them and helping them define the terms that they feel result in interference with performance has been the most helpful tool. Initially, some team members and coaches have been reticent to having such a meeting, but in the end, everyone felt relieved, at least to be able to bring such concerns out in the open. The decisions were not to "forbid" sexual intimacy between teammates—that would have been a useless and an unenforceable rule—but to make sure that friendships and relationships were not exclusive; that is, they were not closed to the rest of the team and did not preclude each of the members from having other friendships and doing activities with other teammates. This was an ongoing process, as we all struggled with ways of dealing with it. Making different room assignments on trips was one way one team agreed to help the situation. I do not claim to have found a solution to this issue, but I would like to see it addressed openly by the sport psychologists. Interventions with coaches must rely heavily on education. Individual support for "stressed-out," isolated coaches is also important. Continuing discussions in open forums, involving all the different parties, is essential.

Summary

Are these gender differences something that a sport psychology consultant should be aware of when working with teams? Of course they are. Issues such as communication, past histories of success and failure, starting status, personal preferences, parenting responsibilities, and relationships and sexual orientations are all commonly manifested problems on teams. How the coach, team members, and the sport psychologist handle these areas will greatly determine the performance of the team and the experience each athlete takes away from this association.

References

Balague, G., Taylor, J., LeScanff, C., & Botterill, C. (1997). The role of the sport psychologist traveling with athletes or teams. *Journal of Applied Sport Psychology, 9,* (Suppl.), S170.

Cahn, S. (1994). *Coming on strong: Gender and sexuality in 20th century women's sport.* Cambridge: Harvard University Press.

Dinkmeyer, D. C., & Losoney, L. E. (1980). *The encouragement book: Becoming a positive person.* Englewood Cliffs, NJ: Prentice Hall.

Griffin, P. (1998). *Strong women, deep closets.* Champaign, IL: Human Kinetics.

Krane, V. (1996). Lesbians in sport: Toward acknowledgment, understanding and theory. *Journal of Sport and Exercise Psychology, 18,* 237-246.

McKay, M., Davis, M., & Fanning, P. (1983). *Messages: The communication skills book.* Oakland, CA: Harbinger Publications.

Messner, M. (1992). *Power at play: Sports and the problem of masculinity.* Boston: Beacon.

Tuffy, S. L. (1996). *Psychological characteristics of male and female athletes and their impact on coach behavior.* Unpublished manuscript.

Vernacchia, R., Balague, G., Yambor, J., & Shaw, T. (1995, September). *Elite athletes and motherhood.* Symposium conducted at the 1995 Association for the Advancement of Applied Sport Psychology Conference, New Orleans.

PART III

PERFORMING SPORT PSYCHOLOGY WITHIN THE TEAM: SPECIFIC SPORTS

CHAPTER 8

Working With Professional Basketball Players

Keith Henschen and David Cook

Abstract

Professional athletes in general and professional basketball players in particular are unique individuals. They are not special people, but rather people with special physical talents who are forced to live a little differently than the rest of us. It is the rare professional athlete who effectively deals with "living-in-the-glass-house." Having stated all of the above, it remains imperative that sport psychologists understand that they are still very much needed by professional team-sport athletes if they are able to deliver services properly. This chapter points out that team interventions are normally not acceptable, coaches are crucial to the success of the sport psychologist, and individual counseling with players and coaches should be the primary method of service delivery. Frequent issues encountered by the sport psychologist are slumps, motivation, use of free time, fragile egos, coaching dynamics, cliques, and the "end-of-the-bench" syndrome. A few other issues that are commonly addressed include dealing with the media, handling success and failure, and handling trades. The chapter concludes with "words of advice" from the authors based on their personal experiences.

Professional athletes in general and professional basketball players in particular are physically gifted and, for the most part, they have been treated as very special people in the societies from which they come. This point is presented only to remind the reader that professional team-sport athletes are frequently considered celebrities (by society and sometimes by themselves) and therefore must be worked with accordingly. All of the various aspects of sport psychology (both applied and clinical) that professionals in our field are taught can be utilized with professional athletes, but should be applied in unique ways.

Professional team-sport members need to be handled by the sport psychologist first and foremost with confidentiality and also with the highest ethical behavior. Professional athletes are people with special physical talents, and they live in their own special world. Professional team-sport athletes are particularly vulnerable to great fan adulation, excessive media pressure, idealistic role-model expectations from the public, and limited private lives. All of this, of course, is the result of their celebrity status. Nevertheless, it is the rare professional athlete who comes naturally equipped to effectively deal with this living-in-a-glass-house environment to which he or she is subjected.

Because of all of the above, it is imperative that sport psychologists understand that they are very much needed by professional team sports—if they can deliver their services properly. Other chapters of this book present excellent material on the ways of, and the importance of, establishing rapport between team-sport athletes and sport psychologists, developing team cohesion, dealing with the emotional aspects of team performance, and working with various professional sports.

It is probably the dream of almost everyone who works in applied sport psychology to eventually have the opportunity to "show their skills" at the professional level of sports. This chapter will share the experiences and reflections of two sport psychology consultants who have worked with successful National Basketball Association (NBA) teams for a number of years. Discussion will center on how to effectively work with these professional athletes (what a consultant can and cannot do), the frequent issues encountered, and suggestions on how to successfully solve some of the problems faced. Generally the authors have provided the following services: group dynamics training, individual counseling, and contributions during the draft process. Frequent problems encountered include counseling players on slumps, motivational issues, and use of free time; handling fragile egos, dealing with coaches; working with cliques; dealing with the end-of-the-bench·syndrome; and helping the players effectively interact with the media.

Team Interventions

Rarely at the professional level will the sport psychologist be called upon to deliver interventions to the entire team. This is not to say that many individuals on a team do not need a particular intervention, but due to coaches' and athletes' attitudes to psychological interventions, team sessions geared to intervention acquisition will rarely be allowed. Group intervention sessions may not be acceptable, but that does not mean that the sport psychologists should not meet with the team regularly. These meetings should be designed to discuss "team issues" and to raise levels of understanding. For example, with a young team, team-cohesion issues become problematic (Carron & Hausenblas, 1998). A team meeting at which we discuss various forms of cohesion and ways to further develop or enhance them is most appropriate. Raising the level of awareness or understanding of an issue by the team members is more effective than just telling them what to do and forcing them to do it. For the most part, professional athletes are mature and want to be treated as such. They all enjoy winning, and if the sport psychologist can link their team success to the principles being presented, then they more than likely will buy into the concept being presented. Other topics frequently of interest from a team perspective are motivational issues, coaching styles, retirement, and dealing with the media.

Working With Coaches

What is presented in this section will be controversial, yet we believe very appropriate and accurate. Team interventions will be neither successful nor accepted by the players unless the coaches are 100% behind the program. If coaches hesitate or disagree in the least with what is being presented by the sport psychologist, then the particular issue is doomed from the onset at the team level. Athletes will judge the importance of all interventions based on the support they receive from the coaching staff—especially the head coach. Therefore, it is our contention that any team intervention should be first presented to the coaching staff and any questions or disagreements be rectified prior to presentation to the team. Any so-called "chink in the armor" or hesitation by the coaches will convey a negative message to the athletes in terms of the importance of the concept. This is not to imply that a good, thorough discussion of an issue is undesirable, but rather, that somewhere near the conclusion of the team meeting, a coach (preferably the head coach) should voice support for what is being presented.

A side note to this is that team administrators (general managers, personnel directors, etc.) should not be asked to support what the sport psychologist is presenting to the coaches and athletes. At the professional level there is normally a common bond or mutual respect between players and coaches; team administrators are frequently not considered a part of this relationship. Players look upon owners and team officials negatively, so ideas and interventions to be employed should not be associated with this segment of the organization.

Although team interventions are infrequently applied at the professional level, an applied sport psychology consultant can provide significant contributions in three direct areas and one indirect area. The three direct areas include group dynamics, individual counseling, and assessment during the draft process. The indirect area is an extensive referral system.

Group Dynamics

Frequently, teams that are winning have more cohesion or "chemistry" than do those that are losing. Nevertheless, cohesion among athletes and with the coaching staff is an ever-present challenge. At the professional level, task cohesion is far more important than social cohesion. It is often assumed that because these basketball players are professionals, they will naturally act with maturity and character. However, this is often a false assumption. Physical ability alone rarely transforms an athlete into a professional and mature team member. The difficult challenge a sport psychology consultant is faced with is that professional players are resistant to working on chemistry as a group. So the consultant normally only works with individuals to achieve group cohesion. This is an unusual way to work towards this goal, but the situation dictates it. The consultant must be highly aware of the cliques within the team. Mentoring of young players by the veteran players is an ideal way to facilitate cohesion; however, some players are resistant to this process. Group dynamics is achievable without team meetings, but achieving such a goal takes patience and creativity on the part of the consultant (Carron, Spink, & Prapavessis, 1997).

Individual Counseling

Many of the problems faced by professional basketball players are best addressed one-on-one and away from the basketball environment. These problems will be discussed later in this chapter. One overriding observation is that it is difficult for highly paid professional basketball players to admit to a need for help—especially in the psychological area. Teaching NBA players psychological interventions or handling problematic issues is best accomplished away from the court (i.e., in your professional office or in the quiet recesses of a secluded restaurant where the players are not likely to be noticed). Incidentally, the consultant should always "pick up the tab," no matter how much a player earns, because this seems to help build the relationship. We have an arrangement with the teams with which we work to have expense accounts cover the cost of these types of meetings. This arrangement has worked very well.

Physical giftedness of a player is not generally related to "mental giftedness." The common interventions of relaxation, concentration training, self-talk, imagery training, and mental routines are needed by many NBA players. Remember: NBA players are not exceptional in all areas of performance; they are just people with special physical talent.

The Draft Process

Another major contribution a sport psychology consultant can make is to become involved in the drafting process. It is not our job to assess athletic ability; instead, we should concentrate on determining how a prospective player would fit into the team and if the player could adjust or respond effectively to the type of coaching currently available. To accomplish this end, we normally attend two of the three scouting combines and psychologically test the perspective players as well as extensively interview them. Due to great investment (monetarily) a team has in a player, it is imperative that the player fit in with the team and be able to respond favorably to the coaching. A poor draft choice is devastating to a team's productivity and cohesive atmosphere. Although different teams use a variety of psychological assessment instruments (ranging from the highly clinical to pop psychology), we have had success using Ogilvie and Greene's Learning Styles and Competitive Styles Profiles (Ogilvie & Greene, 1997). These two instruments provide invaluable information.

Referral System

The indirect area where sport psychology consultants can make a significant contribution to the team, as was previously mentioned, is to know their limits and to supplement their expertise with an extensive referral system. If the consultant is successfully accepted by the players, coaches, and management, these individuals may request help with other psychological issues, those that are beyond the consultant's training. It is very common to be asked to help in family issues (i.e., marriage counseling, general counseling), behavioral problems (i.e., panic attacks, depression), or clinical issues (i.e., bipolar disorders, suicide). It is critical to have an established referral network from day one. It is wise not to become deeply involved in clinical issues, because this may confuse the consultant's role in the mind of the athlete and the team. One should work only in the areas where one is truly an expert. We say this because if a consultant ever makes a mistake, his or her credibility with the player or coach involved is likely to be compromised. Players will look to consultants for help in finding a solution to their problems, but not necessarily in providing the solution personally.

Frequent Issues Faced in the NBA

When working with an NBA team, sport psychology consultants will encounter a number of problem areas that include, but are not limited to, the following: slumps, motivation, free time, fragile egos, coaching dynamics, cliques, the end-of-the-bench syndrome, and crisis intervention.

Slumps

There is nothing more frustrating to a professional athlete or team than to encounter and endure a performance slump. Every athlete and team will be faced with this psychological barrier at one time or another. We identify this as a psychological problem because our experience has shown that slumps initially caused by technical or physical reasons will eventually affect the mind-set of the player or team. Dealing with a slump can test a consultant's counseling expertise. This task is extremely difficult, because the consultant will have to reconstruct the players' or team's pattern of thinking. Most athletes and teams will attempt to overcome a slump by trying harder, thus thinking more. The opposite is required to break out of most slumps. By the time the consultant is approached to provide help, the athlete or team often has tried everything in their repertoire. Often we are the last resort. Also, by the time we enter the picture, frustration is at such a high level that reality is in the distance. The media also add pressure, and often the coaching staff loses confidence in the player or team, and they can even begin talking about trading some of the team members.

The first step in dealing with a slump is to converse with the coaches to make sure that the athlete or team is not doing something fundamentally or physically incorrect. There are times when the coach believes a technical change is needed, whereas the consultant believes a mental adjustment would suffice. It is best to be patient and not challenge the coach's authority. Eventually the consultant will help solve the issue, but always on the coach's terms. The consultant must never challenge the coach's authority, or the consultant will be out the door in a flash. If the team's techniques are still correct, then we can proceed. We start with mitigating the frustration instead of focusing on the outcome. Then we simplify the issue by lessening the amount of thinking and stopping negative self-talk (Vallerand, 1983). We have the players concentrate on a few positive trigger cues, which can help eliminate the inner dialogue and subsequent overanalysis. We keep reinforcing the idea that the players should go back to having fun. When the players return to just playing naturally instead of "trying to make it happen," then the slump will be history.

Motivation

The NBA is a strange game from a reinforcement perspective. Frequently, players are given (guaranteed) millions of dollars before they prove they can play in a league. Due to this financial situation, these players are set for life monetarily (extrinsic motivation) and therefore must focus on the intrinsic reasons for competing to stay on top of their game. It is a challenge to get young players to stay motivated when all their financial concerns are taken care of for life. Imagine having enough money to do anything you want for the rest of your life—it very well could affect your work ethic.

This is often the situation in which the NBA players find themselves. They are young, have plenty of money, and receive a tremendous amount of recognition. So why should they be motivated to work hard and become a better player or a better team? The glamorous lifestyle and enormous financial security can become a curse to immature players instead of a blessing.

The first solution to this problem is to select or trade for ball players who have "heart." There are two components of heart: intrinsic motivation and an unquenchable work ethic. Strangely enough, few players possess both of these characteristics. Some players have a lot of intrinsic drive but lack the work ethic; others work extremely hard, but only for external rewards. Intrinsically motivated players are easier to mold into a cohesive team (Deci & Ryan, 1985;

Weiss & Chaumeton, 1992). The sport psychology consultant is often called upon to work with those players who demonstrate a lack of heart. Here again is an area where one's counseling skills will be tested. The consultant must find out what motivates an individual player and begin from this foundation. The good news is that both intrinsic motivation and a solid work ethic can be developed. It is not easy, but it is possible to learn to have heart. An old adage applies here:

> Question: What do you give a man who has everything?
> Answer: Nothing! You just make him want to have more of what he already has.

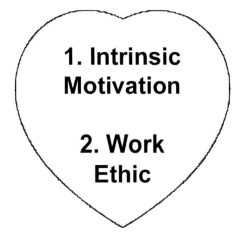

Free Time

This is a fascinating problem faced by all NBA teams. Being a professional basketball player really does not occupy much time. The season is only eight months long, and during the season, practice is only a couple of hours a day. How to deal with all this free time in a constructive manner is frequently a major issue. If the player is married then free time becomes less of an issue when at home, but time on the road is still problematic. Idle time is time to get in trouble, especially for young, energetic, vulnerable millionaires. We counsel all of our players to develop a pattern of time management while on the road. We encourage them to engage in stimulating activities while traveling in other cities. They can visit historical sites, museums, and cultural exhibitions. Endeavors such as reading, movies, and general intellectual pursuits are also advised. It is also important for players to spend time together in small groups while on the road. "Homies" (outside individuals) are discouraged and asked to stay away from the players while they are on the road. This may appear to be a manipulation of a player's personal time—and it probably is—but many players are not equipped to effectively deal with a lot of free time. Many times players will stay in their rooms and sleep, then come to the game and perform with no energy. The important point here is to get the players to stay as active on the road as they would be if they were home.

Fragile Egos

Probably one of the most frequent problems a sport psychologist must deal with is the ego of the various players. There is nothing fair about professional basketball. There is a hierarchy of treatment in the NBA. Superstars are treated differently, both on and off the floor. Some players get paid more, receive more recognition, get more playing time, and are treated differently by the coaching staff as well as the team management. This becomes even more difficult because all NBA athletes have been stars in the colleges and universities where they have previously played basketball. Having been stars, they have been treated accordingly, which frequently conditions their self-concepts as well as their egos. Many athletes have become accustomed to being treated preferentially, and most people enjoy special treatment. However, many have trouble once the "specialness" ends.

The following is a story from personal experience: A young rookie (first-round draft choice) was obviously receiving a great deal of attention (mostly negative) from the coaching staff early in the season. At lunch with the sport psychology consultant, he revealed that "he felt like he had a target on his back" and he wondered out loud if he would ever do anything right. His talent, of course, was exceptional. In college he was physically superior to his competition, and his coaches very seldom criticized him. Contributing to the problem was that he was now placed in the starting lineup because of an injury to another, more experienced player. The coaching staff was concerned because he had so much to learn in a short period of time, and due to his nonchalant personality, he appeared to be loafing at times. He said, "I don't think the coaches like me."

As they talked about his situation, the consultant offered a few observations to the player. First, he needed to remove his ego from the situation and concentrate on the task at hand—learning the offensive plays and also positioning himself properly on defense. Second, he had to quit taking things personally. The consultant related to him that the coaches thought very highly of him, but wanted to make sure he was properly prepared. The consultant also pointed out that he was playing with two perennial "all stars" and two other very seasoned veterans. Who did he think the coaches would naturally be watching the majority of the time? The consultant made two other suggestions: (a) the player should be more demonstrative and energetic on defense and (b) ask questions when he was confused. The young player took this advice and in a couple of weeks was much more comfortable concerning his perception of the treatment he was receiving. He was leaving his ego at home, and his performance as a team member improved.

Counseling of the players' concerns and perceptions of mistreatment is an ongoing process. If these perceptions are not resolved, then jealousy, dislike, and deeply hurt feelings are the consequences. We talk very frankly with players about their egos as well as the inequitable dealings in the NBA. There is nothing fair about the NBA system, so it is counterproductive to perpetuate this façade. The very nature of professional sports is discriminatory. Stars receive more of everything. Players with fragile egos need to be helped to focus on their performances in the name of the team and their personal work ethics, rather than fall into the trap of comparison. Providing a realistic perspective for the athlete is often effective. Role players and reserves are a fact of life in the NBA, and all the hurt feelings and frustrations will not alter this situation. Players need to refocus on what they need to do to improve their situations and to possibly move into the more preferred or favored level. In essence, the second-string players are being compensated greatly to endure this unfair treatment. This may seem harsh, but is that not the nature of competition? Fragile egos can destroy team cohesion if not dealt with openly and immediately. Encouraging the coaching staff to define roles and to reinforce each player in his or her team role is one way to build team unity.

Coaching Dynamics

As sport psychology consultants working in the NBA, it has become clear to us that not only the athletes need attention but also the coaching staffs, which normally consist of 5 to 7 individuals. This is a small group, but nevertheless it is still a group. As might be expected, these small groups have problems similar to those of the actual players. Counseling the staff is delicate work because, here again, there is a hierarchy of importance in the coaching staff.

In reality, some coaches are more important than others, but each has his or her function. The sport psychologist must befriend all the coaches. The most important information we have provided to the coaches we work with are conflict-resolution techniques. Sometimes we are even called upon to facilitate these volatile conflict sessions. Remember: Coaching staffs are really just small groups who are prone to the same pressures and problems as any other small group. They should be handled like other groups. Coaches at the professional level live in a bubble where the world revolves around their sport. They often have enormous power and out-of-balance egos. Bringing to them perspective, penetrating their bubble, and helping them emerge beyond this trap are important tasks that we can perform. However, coaches may feel threatened by our insight, because everyone else around them participates in their bubble world.

Cliques

In any group of more than four to six people, cliques will naturally form. Coaching staffs and the actual team will both have cliques. Cliques in and among themselves are natural, but some can become detrimental to the productivity of the team or staff. The sport psychologist should be aware of the existence of these subsets and monitor them constantly. Knowledge of their changing dynamics is essential to maintain task cohesion.

End-of-the-Bench Syndrome

It is inevitable that by the conclusion of the season only 7 or 8 players are really getting a consistent chance to play during the important parts of the games. Even though 12 players are necessary to practice efficiently, not all of these players are crucial for game performance. Misery loves company. Those 3 or 4 players who are practicing but not getting a chance to demonstrate their abilities during the games have a tendency to bond together and easily become a negative clique. They almost become a small team within the overall team. Frequently, their behaviors mimic each other, and they display their dissatisfaction at not playing by acting disinterested in the team's performance. They become highly paid spectators instead of high-energy substitutes or supporters. The sport psychologist must be actively involved with this group by constantly interacting with them and encouraging them to work hard and provide support for those players who are getting playing time. Usually, the end-of-the-bench syndrome is displayed by young players (who don't know any better) and by veteran players at the end of their careers (who do know better but no longer really care). Young players who mistakenly fall into this syndrome are shortening their careers and doing damage to their reputations (not to mention to the team cohesion). Candid counseling with these players is called for by the sport psychologist. Coaches and management have long memories when it comes to the negative behaviors caused by the end-of-the-bench syndrome. Players need to be aware that their actions are being monitored even when they are not playing. Staying focused on the game is the one way to mitigate the effects of this syndrome.

Other Considerations

There are a few additional considerations that the sport psychology consultant will need to address on a continual basis. Dealing with the media, handling success and failure, and working through trades and free agency are three areas that can cause team problems if not dealt with effectively.

Dealing With the Media

The press is simultaneously a blessing and a curse. It provides a tremendous amount of publicity (marketing) at virtually no cost to the team or the players. It is a curse because the media have shaped this game and continue to exert undue influence on this sport. The overwhelming culprit is, of course, television. Television now dictates how and when the games are played, as well as who will be anointed as the super stars and which teams are anointed as being the most attractive.

Again, a story from personal experience: A very talented player came to me and asked for suggestions on how to conduct a better interview with the media. He had been interviewed a number of times and did not like how he responded to some of the questions, especially those with dealing with other players or his views on matters outside the actual game. He and the consultant discussed the specific things in the interview that actually made him uncomfortable. His response was that looking and talking to that "ugly black microphone" and then having to stop and collect his thoughts before answering made him look less intelligent.

Two suggestions were offered to him by the consultant: (1) He should look the interviewer right in the eyes and carry on a conversation with just that individual. This was practiced a few times in the dressing room with the consultant using his hand (covered with a black sock) as a microphone. (2) The player should also structure the interview so that he felt more in control. He was to give interviews only in the dressing room after a game, not in the hall on the way to the dressing room or on the playing floor. He was also to tell the media that he would talk about only his play and the game and not other issues. This was to be made clear before the microphone was turned on. If a media person violated this agreement, the player was simply to say, "I have no comment on that," and end the interview.

I can't express just how proud I was of this player during an interview after a play-off game. When he saw me watching his interview, he asked the interviewer to turn off the microphone for a second and said to me, "You know, this is starting to be fun." He then resumed the interview. He was now in control instead of the microphone.

There are two aspects that need to be discussed when dealing with the press: first, helping the athletes handle the media and, second, discussing the role the sport psychologist should have in relation to the press. Most basketball players entering the NBA have limited experience in dealing with the media even though they were big fish in the sea at their university. The onslaught of the NBA media is exhausting. New players may not understand that the press has a job to do and will be their friend one day, but will tear them apart the next day if their performance is less than excellent. The media report the news, no matter if it is good or not so good. They will report the seamy side of sports more frequently than the positive aspects because that side is deemed more newsworthy. Athletes are seldom taught how to conduct interviews, when to talk to the press, and how to manipulate the media to their advantage. As sport psychology consultants, we are often asked by team management to discuss media issues with players and to suggest dos and don'ts on dealing with the press. We emphasize that the press should be spoken to only when the player is composed, never emotional. Few players effectively interview before or after emotionally charged contests. Saying nothing is often better than giving a poor interview. Speaking into a microphone is a skill that must be perfected. Players are also encouraged not to read the papers or listen to radio and television sports talk shows.

The second important aspect of dealing with the press is the role of the sport psychology consultant with the media. Our contention is that, whenever possible, the sport psychologist should stay in the background and avoid the press. It is a good practice to avoid places where the media normally perform their job. After practices during the season and especially during the play-offs, the media will attempt to interview players, coaches, and the medical staff. Consultants should avoid the area where the media congregate. Also, after the game, the NBA league rules state that a team has 10-15 minutes in their locker room when the media are not allowed to be present. This is when the coaches talk to the team and then the players vent their emotions. After this period, the press is allowed into the locker room for 20 minutes for interviews. We advise the sport psychologist to attend the postgame session with the coaches and players, then exit before the locker room is opened to the press. The sport psychology consultant should be a resource, not part of the show. The easiest way to undermine your credibility with players and coaches is to be quoted in the media making specific statements about players on the team or to always be present when the media are there. Players and coaches will notice if a consultant is a "camera hound." Consultants should be nice to the press, but do not go out of their way to provide access to themselves.

Dealing With Success and Failure

In any realm of competition, there will be team members who experience great success and also those who feel as if they have failed. It is important to help athletes maintain a healthy perspective. The season is long and draining (seven months plus the play-offs). Ups and downs are natural consequences of the length and intensity of NBA competition. Success is something most NBA players expect because that is what they have been conditioned to have most of their competitive lives. They are the best of the best and expect to remain so. Failure, on the other hand, is much more difficult to deal with because it is a relatively new experience. Let us provide a recent scenario to illustrate this point:

Another personal story: After a recent play-off game, I received a frantic telephone call from a player's wife. She said her husband had not come home from a game. She was very concerned because this behavior was out of the ordinary for him. He had been under a lot of pressure to perform well by the media, coaching staff, and his teammates. He so wanted to play well that he did just the opposite. He played possibly the worst game of his professional career, and the coach was particularly hard on him (orally) in front of his teammates in the locker room. After the game the player just disappeared. Once the spouse had contacted me, I then called the player's agent to see if the player had talked to him. Fortunately he had. The agent said the player was very dis-traught and needed time to sort out his emotions. I then called the wife and explained where he was (just driving around) and that he was fine. I also assured her that he was not a threat to himself. I asked her to have him call me when he came home. He did call me about 2:30 am, and we set up a breakfast meeting. At breakfast, we discussed his feelings as well as his actions. We worked through his anger and embarrassment and then jointly developed a future plan of action that he should follow. He seemed to be relieved that his emotions were now under control and that he had a plan to follow. Later that day I sat with the head coach and explained what had happened the previous night. He was still upset with the performance of the player but wanted to talk to him. The coach wanted the player to understand that he was critical of the performance of the player, not the player. Once they had their meeting and the player understood the coach's position, the issue was resolved.

Failure is hard to take and should never be readily accepted, but it is some-thing that must be contended with in an appropriate manner if the team per-formance is to improve.

Handling Trades

It is inevitable that trades will occur on all NBA teams. It is our position that we do not want to know who is on the "trading block." If the sport psychol-ogist is aware of who is being traded, then this may subconsciously influence the manner in which the consultant deals with this player. Trades are a natural part of the basketball business, but they necessitate a reconstruction of the team chemistry. When a player is added or subtracted from a team, the group dynamics immediately change, and this is when the sport psychology consult-ant must go to work. The team will need to return to the initial stage of group development (forming) and then once again progress through the other stages (storming, norming, and performing). It is wise to inform the coaches and players about what is happening. If they know what to expect, then they can adjust more quickly (Tuckman, 1965).

Words of Advice

Having worked with NBA teams and players for a number of years, we would like to leave you (the reader) with a few gems of wisdom garnered from our experiences:

1. During practices and shoot-arounds, observe the coach/athlete relationships and pick up on learning styles issues.

2. Relationship building is 90% of our challenge (us with them). To work effectively with a player and/or team it may take two years of trust and relationship building.

3. Get to know the athletic trainers—they know everything about the team.

4. If possible, work with the superstars to help them with perspective. They are forced into virtual isolation because they are constantly hounded by adoring fans and the media. Their daily lives are less than normal.

5. Coaching changes are inevitable, but they are traumatic and cause turmoil. Be ready to take a leading role with the team during the process, but then a backseat until you develop trust with the new coaches.

6. Be aware that the owners and team management are constantly receiving letters from those who want your job. These job searchers will promise to do miracles with free-throw shooting, concentration, etc. Instead of becoming defensive and labeling others as quacks, demonstrate your expertise by discussing the fallacies and credibility of their promises.

7. The sport psychology consultant must have heart, maintain perspective, and never jeopardize personal families to "hang with" an NBA team. You must stand above it all and have a great vantage point.

Summary

Working in the NBA has been professionally and personally rewarding. It is not easy because it is vastly different from working with athletes and teams at any other level. Many of the problems consultants will encounter are identical to those at other levels, but the manner of attacking these issues is different. Professional basketball players are not special people, rather people with special physical talents. They are not what the general population thinks they are. They are just people who have the same needs, problems, desires, and emotions as do other human beings. The problem is this is not what society expects, so players are forced to present an image in public that is not really them. The challenge to the sport psychologist is to get to know the real players. Sport psychologists can contribute in a variety of ways: fostering group dynamics, providing individual counseling, being involved in the drafting process, and having an extensive referral system. NBA players are not normal athletes, but they will still demonstrate a number of common problems that all athletes experience. These are the issues commonly faced by the sport psychologist: slumps, motivational problems, positive utilization of free time, fragile egos, and cliques. There are also a few issues that are specific to professional basketball players and teams: coping with the end-of-the-bench syndrome, dealing with the media, handling success and failure, and working through trades.

Here are a few words of advice for those of you who find yourself working with professional basketball teams. First, be a professional, not a fan. You will compromise effectiveness if you act like a fan. Players want your expertise not your adulation. Second, be yourself around the players and coaches. They will test you to see if you are real. Pass the test. Most athletes can spot a phony from a mile away. Finally, stay in the background and be a resource. Deflect the press and recognition as much as possible to the athletes and coaches. Your presence is to be seen and felt not by the media, but by the team.

References

Carron, A. V., & Hausenblas, H. A. (1998). *Group dynamics in sport* (2nd ed.). Morgantown, WV: Fitness Information Technology.

Carron, A. V., Spink, K. S., & Prapavessis, H. (1997). Team building and cohesiveness in the sport and exercise setting: Use of indirect interventions. *Journal of Applied Sport Psychology, 9,* 61-72.

Deci, E. L., & Ryan, R. M. (1985). *Intrinsic motivation and self-determination in human behavior.* New York: Plenum.

Ogilvie, B., & Greene, D. (1997). *Mental skills inventory.* Los Gatos, CA: Pro Mind Institute.

Tuckman, B. W. (1965). Development sequence in small groups. *Psychological Bulletin, 63,* 384-399.

Vallerand, R. J. (1983). On emotion in sport: Theoretical and social psychological perspectives. *Journal of Sport Psychology, 5,* 197-215.

Weiss, M. R., & Chaumeton, N. (1992). Motivational orientation in sport. In T. S. Horn (Ed.), *Advances in sport psychology* (pp. 61-100). Champaign, IL: Human Kinetics.

CHAPTER 9

Improving Concentration Skills in Team-Sport Performers: Focusing Techniques for Soccer Players

Aidan Moran

Abstract

Concentration, or the ability to focus mental effort on what is most important in any situation while ignoring distractions, is widely regarded as a vital determinant of athletic success at all levels of competition. What psychological mechanisms underlie this skill? Why do sport performers seem to "lose" their focus so easily? What should they concentrate on in competitive situations, and how can they be trained to improve their attentional skills in practice? The purpose of this chapter is to provide some answers to these questions by using research findings from psychology as well as practical examples from the team sport of soccer. Following a brief review of the nature and importance of concentration in sport, an attempt is made to explain why athletes tend to "lose" it through distractibility. Then, after some theoretical principles of concentration have been specified, five practical focusing techniques are illustrated in the case of soccer players. The final section of the chapter summarizes the main theoretical and practical implications of concentration skills training in sport performers.

"I think the concentration went a little bit at times." (Alex Ferguson, manager of Manchester United after a defeat by Bayern Munich in the quarter-final of the European Cup in April 2001, cited in "Reds Boss," 2001, pp. 94-95)

It is October 9, 1999, and the last round of qualifying matches for the Euro 2000 international football tournament is taking place. In Skopje, Macedonia, as the final match in Group 8 is in the third minute of "injury time," the Republic of Ireland team is leading Macedonia by one goal to nothing (1-0) and heading for a victory that will ensure automatic qualification for the championship finals. The referee looks at his watch and decides that there are 10 seconds to go. Suddenly, a corner kick is awarded to the home team. As the ball arches into the penalty area, none of the Irish players notices a Macedonian defender who, having timed his run into the box perfectly, heads the ball powerfully into the Irish net. Goal! An elementary defensive error has cost the Republic of Ireland automatic qualification for Euro 2000. After the match, the recriminations begin. How can international soccer players suddenly forget to "mark up" for a corner kick? After all, a golden rule in the game when defending against set pieces is to "pick up" and shadow opponents as closely as possible. When players become tired, lapses of attention are inevitable, and as the final whistle approaches, weary players often "look after the man nearest to them and tell everyone else to pick up the runner. The result is that everyone stands around waiting for the ball" (Townsend, 1999, p. 45). Clearly, it is precisely this problem of "ball watching" that unhinged the Irish defense in Skopje. Not surprisingly, research suggests that such mental lapses are more likely to occur towards the end, rather than at the beginning, of matches. Indeed, more goals are scored in the final 15 minutes of a game than at any other time-period in a soccer match ("Evening Herald," 2000).

One explanation for this end-of-match vulnerability is that mental effort is required to maintain alertness, and "as fatigue sets in, concentration wanders and more mistakes are made" (Maynard, 1998, p. 25). Of course, such physical fatigue is understandable in view of the fact that outfield players in soccer cover an estimated ten km during the course of a game (Reilly, 1999). Exacerbating the problem of fatigue is the possibility that players tend to lose their "focus" at this stage of the game by thinking too far ahead. Specifically, it is well known that in the final seconds of a game, some footballers begin to make figurative victory speeches instead of dealing with the task at hand. It is precisely this attentional problem that Patrick Vieira, the French international soccer star, referred to when trying to explain how Arsenal lost the 2001 British FA Cup Final to Liverpool by conceding two goals in the last few minutes of the match. As he said, "Maybe we were too confident in ourselves because we were winning 1-0" FA Cup Final, cited in O'Neill, 2001, p. 3). Taken together, these two incidents involving the Republic of Ireland and Arsenal offer compelling evidence that a wandering mind can mean the difference between success and failure in soccer at the highest level. This principle was acknowledged by the Birmingham City defender Kenny Cunningham, who observed that "The biggest difference between club and international football is the concentration level. There are times after international games when physically you could be tired but mentally you're shattered. At times, you've no voice left and maybe a pounding headache. Playing against world-class players is difficult—one lapse in concentration can cost you at this level" (1999, p. 27).

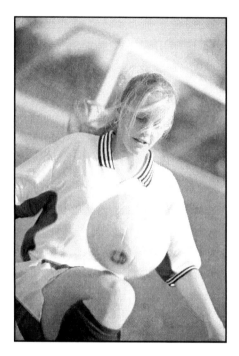

Understanding how concentration is maintained and broken can help coaches keep players on track.

What exactly is "concentration" anyway? Why do athletes "lose" it so easily despite their best intentions? What should they focus on in competitive situations? How can they be trained to improve their concentration skills in practice? The purpose of this chapter is to provide some answers to these and other questions raised by the study of concentration processes in athletes.

The chapter is organized into three sections, as follows. The first section explains the nature and importance of concentration and suggests possible reasons for sport performers' tending to "lose it" so easily. This section will also include a brief analysis of typical distractions encountered in the team sport of soccer, the most popular game in the world. The next section will be devoted to the theory and practice of concentration skills training in athletes. In particular, following the presentation of a number of psychological principles of concentration, the section will describe and illustrate five practical focusing techniques that are used commonly by soccer players. The final section of the chapter will consider some theoretical and practical implications of research on concentration skills training in team-sport performers.

The Nature and Importance of Concentration

In cognitive psychology, concentration is studied as part of the mind's attention system. For over a century, the term attention has had at least three different meanings. Let us now consider each of these interpretations as well as the metaphors with which they are associated.

First, and most frequently, attention has been used as a synonym for "concentration," or the conscious experience of exerting mental effort when perceiving information selectively. For example, a goalkeeper facing a penalty kick concentrates by focusing exclusively on the opponent's run up to the ball in an attempt to guess the likely direction of the shot. This understanding of the term emerges from a "spotlight" metaphor of attention (see review by Fernandez-Duque & Johnson, 1999)—the view that attention resembles a mental light-beam that can illuminate a given target located either in the external world around us or in the subjective domain of our own thoughts and feeling. In accordance with this metaphor, Schmid and Peper (1998) define concentration as the ability to "focus one's attention on the task at hand and thereby not be disturbed or affected by irrelevant internal and external stimuli" (p. 316). In their view, concentration refers to the ability to focus mental effort on what is most important in any situation. To illustrate, consider the selective attentional skills of a champion sprinter, Michael Johnson, the ten-time world gold medallist and the first person to win the 400m event in successive Olympic Games: "I have learned to cut out all the unnecessary thoughts ... on the track. I simply concentrate. I concentrate on the tangible—on the track, on the race, on the blocks, on the things I have to do. The crowd fades away and the other athletes disappear, and now it's just me and this one lane" (cited in Miller, 1997, p. 64). This quotation highlights the benefits of achieving a "focused" mental state in which there is no difference between what one is thinking and what one is doing. Interestingly, it is only relatively recently that sport psychologists have begun to explore empirically the question of precisely what cues athletes should focus on during a competition (see Mallett & Hanrahan, 1997).

Although the spotlight metaphor of attention is historically important and intuitively appealing, it has certain limitations as a heuristic device. For example, it is potentially misleading because it implies that events that occur "outside" the hypothetical area illuminated by the attentional beam (e.g., unconscious processes in the "darkness" of the mind) are unimportant, but modern cognitive research shows that unconscious factors can affect attentional processes significantly. For example, repeated implicit exposure to a stimulus "primes" the attentional system to recognize it faster than in control conditions (Reisberg, 2001). In a more mundane example, trying not to think about something may serve only to increase its prominence in our minds (see review by Wenzlaff & Wegner, 2000). Similarly, attempting to suppress a certain thought in a pressure situation (e.g., "Don't miss this penalty" in soccer) may backfire and lead to ironic performance of the unintended action (Wegner, Ansfield, & Pilloff, 1998). Nevertheless, this spotlight metaphor of attention is useful in reminding us that concentration is never really "lost" but merely redirected at some unhelpful or irrelevant target. Interestingly, this insight challenges what some athletes tell us about their attentional experiences. For example, after a defeat in the 1993 French Open tennis championship, Gabriela Sabatini admitted that she had "lost concentration" during her match against Mary-Jo Fernandez at a stage when she needed just one point for victory (when leading in the match by 6-1, 5-1, 40-15) (Thornley, 1993). In passing, it should be noted that the spotlight metaphor of attention has changed significantly in recent years as a result of advances in neuroscientific technology. Specifically, as Fernandez-Duque and Johnson (1999) explained, cognitive researchers have shifted away from the idea that the attentional spotlight illuminates objects in the surrounding visual field and towards the theory that it shines on brain areas instead. Put simply, the spotlight view of attention is now more accurately described as the "spotlight in the brain" metaphor.

A second way in which the term attention can be interpreted is as a form of mental "time-sharing" that enables people to do two or more tasks at the same time without apparent loss of efficiency. This phenomenon is known as "divided attention" and is illustrated in soccer by the extraordinary ability of some players (e.g., Luis Figo, the brilliant Portuguese star) to dribble with the ball while running at full speed and simultaneously scanning the pitch to assess the positions of teammates. The dominant metaphor here is the idea of attention as a limited pool of mental energy that can be allocated to task demands depending on various psychological principles (e.g., the theory of automaticity proposes that the more a task is practiced, the more attentional resources are "freed up" for concurrent activities) (Abernethy, 2001). In other words, Figo's skills require negligible conscious attention mainly because they have been practiced to an extraordinarily high degree.

The third denotation of the term attention is as a form of biological preparation or alertness. To illustrate, a goalkeeper in soccer may endeavor to maintain his or her arousal levels at a high level by pacing up and down on the goal-line while defending against a corner-kick. Again, the key metaphor here is that of "attention as energy." To summarize, the term attention is a multidimensional construct with at least three different meanings pertaining to perception, action, and arousal states.

Now that we have defined attention, let us consider its importance in athletic performance. Briefly, the critical role of concentration in sport is supported by a combination of empirical evidence and anecdotal insights. To illustrate the former, research on the peak performance experiences of athletes shows that they tend to do their best when they are totally focused on the task at hand (Jackson, 1995). Thus according to Jackson and Csikszentmihalyi (1999), concentration is "a critical component and one of the characteristics of optimal experience mentioned most often" (p. 25). The state of mind engendered by this total absorption in the present task is epitomized by a quotation from Pele, a triple World Cup winner with Brazil and arguably the best soccer player of all time. Commenting on his most memorable performance, he reported that "I felt I could run all day without tiring, that I could dribble through any of their team or all of them, that I could almost pass through them physically" (cited in Jones, 1995, p. 12). Augmenting such research on peak performance experiences are studies of the effects of various attentional strategies on athletic performance in endurance events (e.g., marathon running). For example, the use of "associative" techniques, whereby athletes pay attention explicitly to bodily signals (e.g., heartbeat, respiratory signals, and muscular sensations), is linked significantly with faster performance in running (Masters & Ogles, 1998) and swimming (Couture, Jerome, & Tihanyi, 1999). Similarly, Mallett and Hanrahan (1997) discovered that sprinters who had been trained to use race plans that involved deliberately focusing on task-relevant cues ran faster than when performing in baseline (control) conditions. Apart from such studies, a wealth of anecdotal testimonials to the importance of concentration is available from top athletes as well as from sport psychologists. For example, Teddy Sheringham, the former England soccer star who was voted FA footballer of the year in 2001, revealed that he had learned from the former German international striker Jurgen Klinsmann that "you have to concentrate all the time so when a chance comes you're going to take it" (cited in Lovejoy, 1995, p.19). In the realm of sport science, Abernethy (2001) claimed that "it is difficult to imagine that there can be anything more important to the learning and performance of sports skills than paying attention to the task at hand" (p. 53). In summary, empirical research and anecdotal data confirm the vital role that concentration plays in sport performance.

Why Do Soccer Players "Lose" Their Concentration? Exploring Mental Lapses

Earlier, it was noted that concentration may be defined as the focusing of mental effort on sensory or mental events. As indicated previously, it has been likened to a mental spotlight that we shine at things in which we are interested. What happens if our mental beam dwells on factors that are not relevant to the task at hand? In such circumstances, our concentration will probably be disrupted, and we will become "distracted." Thus, most concentration problems in sport arise because performers fail to pay attention to the "right" cues. For example, a soccer player may make mistakes in a match because he or she is trying to impress a close relative on the sidelines or a scout from another club rather than focusing only on the events taking place on the pitch.

Although distractions come in all shapes and sizes, they may be distinguished in terms of their origins. Thus psychologists propose a distinction between "external" and "internal" distractions (see review in Moran, 1996). "External" distractions consist of environmental factors that divert our attention away from its intended target. In soccer, a myriad of such factors exist. Here are some of them:

- Encountering high noise levels and disruptive crowd behavior (e.g., teams visiting the Turkish football club, Galatasaray, in the Ali Sami Yen stadium in Istanbul have complained of being greeted by throngs of hostile supporters letting off fireworks and waving banners bearing such messages as "Welcome to hell"!),
- Detecting sudden movements from other players in one's peripheral vision (e.g., as happens when jostling occurs among players in a crowded penalty area),
- Being deliberately prevented by opponents from "tracking" the flight of the ball (e.g., at corner kicks, attackers often stand beside the goalkeeper in order to obstruct his or her view of the incoming ball),

- Playing with variations in pitch conditions (e.g., some teams are known to reduce the width of their pitch before matches against teams that play with specialist "wingers"),

- Noticing that substitutes from one's team are "warming up" on the sidelines,

- Succumbing to provocation and "gamesmanship" from one's opponents.

This last problem occurs whenever players use strategic behavioral ploys in an effort to "psych out" their adversaries by attempting to disrupt their concentration (see Table 1).

> ## Gamesmanship, or the art of "winding up," provoking, and/or distracting opponents in an effort to gain some competitive advantage, is rampant in soccer. Below are some examples of this tactic.

"Diving," or pretending to have been fouled during a tackle from an opponent. This practice is prevalent among forwards who seek penalties by falling over theatrically in their opponents' penalty areas. This offense is now punishable by a caution (or "yellow card").
"Shirt-pulling," jostling, or other forms of physical obstruction are commonly encountered when players await free kicks or corner kicks. Usually, this type of gamesmanship is difficult to detect and hence remains largely unpunished.
Verbal abuse ("sledging"/"trash talking") or taunting and insulting opponents (often using racist remarks) is practiced frequently in the game (Selvey, 1999; White, 1999).
Nonverbal "psych outs" are common. For example, in a UEFA cup-match in 1999 between Hapoel Tel Aviv and Glasgow Celtic, a penalty was awarded to the Scottish team. As the kick was about to be taken, the Israeli goalkeeper strode up to the penalty-taker and stared at him for a few seconds, presumably in an effort to upset his concentration ("Evening Herald," 1999). Likewise, Bruce Grobbelar, former Liverpool goalkeeper, used to try to distract penalty-takers by wobbling his knees vigorously just as they were about to strike the ball.
Physical intimidation is widely practiced in soccer. Using this ploy, a player may tackle an opponent illegally or overvigorously early in a tackle in an effort to make him or her more hesitant for the remainder of the game.
Provocative tactics include spitting at opponents (e.g., Holland's Frank Rijkaard was sent off for spitting at Germany's Rudi Voller in the World Cup finals) and pinching them on the scalp while pretending to lift them to their feet after they have fallen in tackles (allegedly encountered by George Best, the former Manchester United star).

Table 1. "Psyching out" opponents: Gamesmanship in soccer

Fortunately, such reprehensible ploys have been increasingly detected and punished by the football authorities in recent years. For example, the Dutch international defender Michael Reiziger was censured for revealing on his Web site how he had planned to provoke Ireland's Roy Keane during a vital World Cup qualifying match in September 2000 (Irish Times, 2000). As we shall see in the next section, the best response to gamesmanship is to use a simple refocusing technique that points the mental spotlight at the task at hand rather than at the source of the distraction.

By contrast with external distractions, "internal" threats to concentration stem from the vast array of thoughts, feelings, and/or bodily sensations (e.g., pain, fatigue) that impede efforts to concentrate on the job at hand. Typical of such self-generated distractions are speculating about the result of a match before it is over, regretting mistakes made previously, worrying about other people's perceived evaluation of one's performance, and/or experiencing feelings of anxiety or fatigue. Interestingly, Dunn (1999) discovered that four main themes emerged when the worries of ice hockey players were analyzed: (a) fear of failure, (b) apprehension about negative evaluation by others, (c) concern about physical injury, and (d) anxiety about the unknown. Unfortunately, despite such pioneering research, little is known about the nature and operation of other "internal" distractions that hamper athletic performance. This neglect can be attributed to a combination of theoretical and methodological biases. First, for many years (specifically, dating back to the "multistore" model of memory; Atkinson & Shiffrin, 1968) researchers assumed falsely that information "flows" into the mind in only one direction—from the outside world inward. In adopting this model, researchers ignored the possibility that information could travel in the opposite direction, namely, from one's long-term memory into one's current awareness. Fortunately, this oversight has been rectified in recent accounts of memory (Solso, 1998). A second reason for the neglect of internal distractions stems from a methodological bias. Specifically, researchers focused on external distractions simply because they were easier to measure than were self-generated distractors (Moran, 1996).

Unfortunately, as a result of these twin biases, the theoretical mechanisms by which internal distractions disrupt concentration were largely ignored until the work of Wegner (1994). According to him, the mind wanders mainly because we try to control it. To explain, when people try to suppress a thought, they engage in a controlled (conscious) search for thoughts that are different from the unwanted thought. At the same time, however, an automatic (unconscious) search takes place for any signs of the unwanted thought. In other words, the intention to suppress a thought activates an automatic search for that very thought in an effort to monitor whether or not the suppression has been successful. Normally, the conscious intentional system dominates the unconscious monitoring system, but under certain circumstances (e.g., when our working memories are overloaded or when our attentional resources are depleted by fatigue or stress), the ironic system prevails and an "ironic intrusion" of the unwanted thought occurs. Wegner attributes this "rebound" effect to cognitive load. Specifically, although this load is believed to disrupt the conscious mechanism of thought control, it does not interfere with the automatic (and ironic) monitoring system. This theory of mental control is supported by experimental evidence that people who tried to concentrate under a heavy cognitive load ended up memorizing, rather than ignoring, the distracters (Zukier & Hagen, 1978). Such research led Wegner to conclude that "the intention to concentrate creates conditions under which mental load enhances monitoring of irrelevancies" (p. 7). To summarize, Wegner's research helps us to understand why athletes may find it hard to suppress unwanted or irrelevant thoughts when they are anxious. Interestingly, research on thought suppression raises doubts about the validity of "thought stopping" as an intervention technique in sport psychology (e.g., see Bull, Albinson, & Shambrook, 1996; Maynard, 1998). Briefly, this technique requires an athlete to use a trigger word like "stop" to halt worries or other unhelpful thoughts. The problem with this procedure is that trying to suppress a thought when one is anxious is likely to lead to an ironic rebound effect. Thus Wegner, Broome, and Blumberg (1997) found that the attempt to relax in certain stressful situations can have ironic, rebound effects on people's electrodermal responses. In other words, trying to relax can sometimes, ironically, generate unintended anxiety. Given such possibilities, the U.S. National Research Council's Committee on Techniques for the Enhancement of Human Performance urges caution in the use of thought-stopping procedures (Wegner, Eich, & Bjork, 1994).

Improving Concentration Skills: Assessment, Principles, and Techniques

Given the importance of concentration to athletic performance, coaches and sport psychologists have experimented with a variety of techniques that are designed to improve athletes' focusing skills. Before any of these interventions can be applied, however, it is important to clarify a number of diagnostic issues (Simons, 1999).

First, what are the concentration demands of the skill in which improvements are required? Is this task an "open" or "closed" skill? Does it require precise, fine motor movements (e.g., "killing" a ball with one's first touch in soccer), or does it depend more on timing or physical strength (e.g., tackling)? Consultation with an expert coach is essential at this stage.

Second, does the player know what precisely he or she should concentrate on when attempting to perform the skill? This question is often overlooked in one's haste to provide an intervention. Indeed, although coaches regularly exhort players to "concentrate" by shouting at them from the sidelines, they rarely check that players understand what exactly they should be paying attention to in that situation. For example, consider the age-old instruction to "watch the ball." Instead of shouting this phrase repeatedly until it becomes meaningless, coaches should consider experimenting with questions such as "What way was the ball spinning as it came to you?" Or "Did you guess correctly where the ball would land just before the player passed it?" The former question is designed to intensify the player's attention to the ball itself whereas the latter question may encourage the detection of advance cues prior to release of the ball. In both cases, the coach's use of questions rather than commands is likely to stimulate discovery learning on the part of the player (see Whitaker, 1999).

Third, it may be helpful to ask the player to specify the main distractions that he or she typically encounters when attempting to perform the skill in question.

Finally, it is vital for the coach or sport psychologist to evaluate the degree to which motivational issues affect the attentional problem under investigation. To explain, lapses in concentration are sometimes attributable simply to a lack of interest on the part of the performer. If so, the difficulty may be motivational rather than cognitive in nature, and the priority that the player attaches to the task may have to be questioned.

Assuming that these questions have been answered adequately, how can we help players to improve their concentration skills? Based on the famous dictum that "there is nothing so practical as a good theory" (Lewin, 1951, p. 169), here is a theoretically based set of concentration principles along with associated intervention techniques.

Concentration Principles

Based on the relevant empirical research literature (see reviews by Abernethy, Summers, & Ford, 1998; Moran, 1996), at least five theoretical principles of concentration may be identified (see Figure 1).

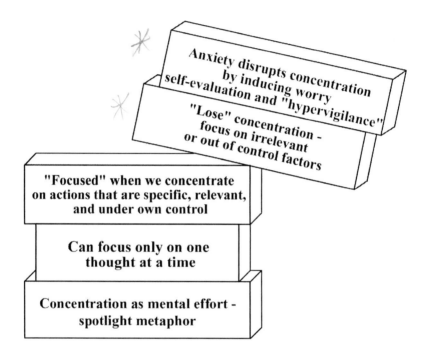

Figure 1. Concentration principles

To begin with, effective concentration requires intentionality and mental effort and is best regarded as the skill of focusing on what is most important in any situation while ignoring distractions. Influenced by the spotlight metaphor, we can interpret concentration as a "beam" of mental energy that we "shine" at things (i.e., stimuli from external or internal sources) in which we are interested. Second, although we are capable of dividing our attention between two or more actions, we can focus consciously on only one thought at a time. This limitation of consciousness is explained in part by the fragility and limited span of the working memory system that regulates our attentional resource (see Logie, 1999). Third, our minds are "focused" optimally when there is no difference between what we are thinking about and what we are doing. In other words, we tend to concentrate most effectively when we direct our attention at actions that are specific, relevant, and under our own control. Fourth, we are said to "lose" our concentration when we pay attention to things that are out of our control, not in the present, or otherwise irrelevant to the task at hand. Finally, anxiety tends to impair our concentration system in several distinctive ways. For example, it engages our limited working memory resources in "worry"—a cognitive activity involving "a chain of thoughts and images (that are) negatively affect laden (and) relatively uncontrollable" (Borkovec, Robinson, Pruzinsky, & DuPree, 1983, p. 10; see also Dunn, 1999). In addition, by elevating our levels of physiological arousal, anxiety tends to restrict the "beam" of our mental spotlight and shift its focus onto self-referential (and usually irrelevant) stimuli. Thus Janelle, Singer, and Williams (1999) found that anxious drivers who participated in a motor-racing simulation were more likely to attend to irrelevant cues than when compared with a baseline condition. Interestingly, these findings were anticipated over four decades ago in Easterbrook's (1959) theory of how "attentional narrowing" can occur in anxiety-provoking situations. Finally, anxiety influences the direction of our attentional focus by encouraging us to dwell on real or imagined personal weaknesses (self-focused attention), potential threats in the environment (thereby inducing a state of "hypervigilance"), and/or on the possible results of what we are doing. In short, anxiety affects the content, direction, and "width" of our concentration beam.

Concentration Techniques

Based on the preceding theoretical principles, a number of practical concentration techniques may be used to promote "focusing" skills in soccer players (see Figure 2; also Moran, 2000). A key feature of these procedures is that they attempt to ensure that the minds of the players are focused on actions that are specific, relevant, and under their own control (Moran, 1996; Moran, 1998).

As is evident from Figure 2, the five concentration techniques to be explained include (a) specifying performance goals, (b) using routines, (c) using trigger words, (d) engaging in mental practice or "visualization," and (e) simulation training.

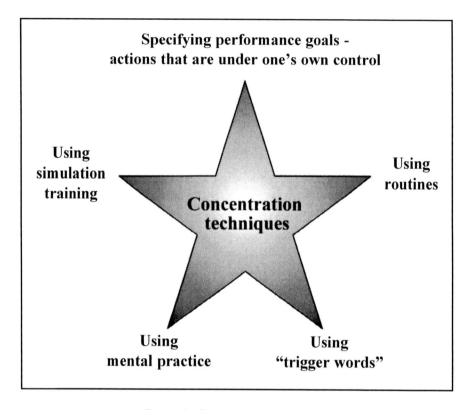

Figure 2. Concentration techniques

Specifying performance goals. Goals are targets or objectives that we strive to achieve. Without them, the energy or "drive" of athletes and players would go to waste. For example, imagine sitting in a car that is being driven around in circles in a parking lot. Although energy is being expended in this movement, one is not actually going anywhere. By analogy, in order to make progress in any sport, athletes need a goal or a signpost to point them in the right direction. That is why goal setting is a useful technique for improving concentration: It signposts appropriate cues for optimal attentional focus. Not all goals are equally effective in enhancing concentration. Thus, if players think too much about "result goals" that are outside their control (e.g., winning a match), they may end up distracting themselves by thinking too far ahead. Accordingly, coaches and sport psychologists recommend that players should concentrate as much as possible on "performance goals"—tasks that are under their control and that can be performed in the immediate present. For example, the secret of maintaining one's concentration when taking a penalty kick is to focus entirely on placing the ball in a particular direction (e.g., just inside the left-hand post), rather than worrying about whether or not the goalkeeper will save it. Interestingly, this principle is supported by research evidence. For example, Jackson and Roberts (1992) discovered that collegiate athletes tended to give their worst performances when they were preoccupied by result goals. Conversely, their best displays coincided with a concern for performance or "process" goals.

To illustrate the use of performance goals to improve concentration, consider the "consecutive passes" drill that is often used in soccer training (Simon & Reeves, 1985). In this exercise, two 7-a-side teams compete against each other in a 15-minute match. The objective, however, is not to score goals but to retain possession of the ball for one's team by completing a series of 8 consecutive passes. The exercise can be made more difficult by raising the criterion number of passes to be achieved (e.g., from 8 to 10) and/or by requiring that players take only two touches on the ball, one to control it and the second to pass it. The purpose of this drill is to train players to concentrate on finding a teammate with a pass rather than playing the ball mindlessly upfield. This type of training is very important in preparing players to retain possession of the ball when defending a lead in pressure situations (e.g., when there are only a few minutes to go and the opposing team is attacking repeatedly).

Using routines. Have you ever noticed that most sport stars follow characteristic or "trademark" sequences of preparatory actions before they perform key skills? For example, in soccer, penalty-takers tend to favor a particular style and distance for the "run up" to their kicks and players taking "throw-ins" often rub their hands on their shirts before gripping the ball—even on dry days. These preferred action sequences are called "preperformance routines" (see also chapter 4 by Lidor and Singer in this book) and are widely practiced by team-sport performers, especially before the execution of "closed" skills (i.e., actions that can be performed without interference from other people). For example, a prepenalty routine in soccer might involve placing the ball on the penalty spot, deciding where one wants to place the shot, taking a set number of steps back, pausing for a second to take a deep breath, and then commencing the run-up to the ball.

At least three types of routines may be identified among soccer players. To begin with, "prematch" routines refer to preferred sequences of actions that players like to follow prior to competitive matches. Included here are "scripts" governing what to do the night before the competition, on the morning of the match, and in the final hours before the game. The second type of routines concerns preperformance actions. Here, the focus is on preparing oneself to perform a closed skill (e.g., a corner kick) during the game. Finally, "postmistake" routines are increasingly apparent. These action sequences are simply ways of putting mistakes in the past and getting on with the task at hand. Accordingly, they are effectively ways of refocusing attention after a mistake has occurred. To illustrate, soccer players are trained to face the ball after a free kick has been awarded against them rather than to dispute the decision with the referee or to blame other players. Clearly, as Arsene Wenger, the manager of the 2001-2 English Premiership champions, Arsenal, observed, "when you argue with the referee you are not concentrating on the game and you lose two or three seconds" (cited in Lacey, 1997, p. 5). Similarly, players may be trained to offer encouragement rather than criticism to teammates who have made mistakes or have been dispossessed by opponents. The value of this routine is that it helps to refocus the player's attention on what he or she can do immediately to correct the mistake (Syer, 1989). Other soccer situations that require players to refocus rapidly include the moments immediately after a goal has been scored or conceded and those that follow stoppages in play as a result of injuries to players.

In general, routines are believed to improve concentration in three main ways. First, they encourage players to develop an appropriate mental "set" for skill execution by helping them to focus their thoughts so that they attend only to task-relevant information. For example, most goalkeepers follow prekick routines to help them to minimize the distractions arising from the jeering that is often directed at them from the supporters of opposing teams. Second, routines ensure that athletes remain focused on the "here and now" rather than on what happened in the past or on what may occur in the future. Finally, routines help players to generate an appropriate mood for competitive performance. In a remark attributed to the famous American psychologist William James, "it is easier to act your way into a feeling than to feel your way into an action." Breaks in play afford useful opportunities for the use of routines. Thus soccer players can use them before goal kicks, throw-ins, and free kicks. Interestingly, there is growing research evidence that routines can improve athletes' concentration and performance. For example, Jackson and Baker (2001) recently conducted a case study of the prestrike routine used by the brilliant Welsh international rugby kicker, Neil Jenkins. They identified such techniques as thought stopping and mental imagery as key components of this player's routine, but they also discovered that contrary to theoretical predictions, Jenkins varied the timing of his prekick behavior as a function of the difficulty of the kick. Other evidence on the efficacy of routines is also available. For example, Crews and Boutcher (1986) compared the performances of two groups of golfers—those who had been given an 8-week training program of swing practice only and those who had participated in a practice-plus-routine program for the same duration. Results revealed that the more proficient golfers benefited more from using routines than did the less skilled players.

One problem with the use of routines, however, is that they may lead to superstitious behavior, but sport psychologists try to distinguish between routines and superstitions on two main grounds. First, they consider the issue of control. A superstition arises from the belief that one's fate is governed by factors outside one's control. A player who uses routines should feel that components of his or her preperformance preparation could be shortened if necessary. By contrast, superstitious rituals tend to lengthen as more and more behavioral links are added to the imaginary chain between action and consequence. A second criterion that may be used to distinguish between routines and rituals concerns the technical role of each behavioral step followed. Whereas each part of a routine should be justifiable logically, the components of a ritual may seem irrational. Unfortunately, despite such neat distinctions, the preshot routines of many footballers are often invested with a superstitious quality.

Using "trigger words" as concentration cues. Most sports performers talk to themselves covertly as they train or compete. Often, athletes tend to be critical of themselves rather than self-congratulatory. Unfortunately, by engaging in such self-criticism, they may end up distracting themselves even further. Therefore, what is required is a set of concise and vivid verbal cues (or "trigger words") that can be used to signal the appropriate attentional focus for a particular game situation. For example, in soccer, a cue word like "keeper" is used to signal that the goalkeeper has decided to come out of goal in an effort to claim a cross. Similarly, the trigger word "away" is often used by goalkeepers to encourage their defenders to head the ball out of danger at free kicks or corner kicks. Similarly, the trigger word "time" is used to signal to a player in possession of the ball that he or she is not about to be challenged by an opponent and has sufficient time to pass the ball to a teammate. Likewise, "hold it" is a useful phrase to remind a player to retain possession until a teammate is in a good position to receive a pass. Also, a phrase like "get tight" is often used by coaches to remind players to shadow their opponents as closely as possible. In general, psychologists recommend that effective trigger words should have four main characteristics (Schmid & Peper, 1998). First, they must be phrased to enable players to focus on positive (i.e., "what to do") rather than negative (i.e., "what to avoid") targets. Second, they should emphasize what needs to be done in the present situation rather than in the future. Third, they should target the process of the skill instead of its outcome. Finally, it may be helpful for trigger words to be written down on cards and made visible to the player during training.

Mental practice. The term mental practice or visualization refers to the systematic use of mental imagery in order to rehearse physical actions. It involves "seeing" and "feeling" a skill in one's imagination before actually executing it (Moran, 1996). Apparently, this technique is widely practiced by soccer players. For example, the former Manchester United star George Best reported using mental imagery as a technique for focusing his mind before matches. Thus he claimed that "the night before a match, I would lie in bed and plot what I was going to do on the field the next day. I used to imagine myself pushing the ball between the legs of the defender who I knew would be marking me, and the next day I would go out and do it" (Best, 1990, p. 28).

Although mental practice has been shown to improve skilled performance (e.g., see review by Driskell, Copper, & Moran, 1994), its status as a concentration technique is uncertain. It appears to work, however, by helping players to form a mental "blueprint" of the sequence of movements that they are trying to learn. For example, a common problem with wingers in football is that they tend to favor one direction when confronted by a defender. Naturally, this tendency (which is probably linked to "handedness" or "footedness") is a liability in a player because it is easily detected by opposing coaches in scouting reports. A possible solution to this difficulty is to encourage players to visualize themselves receiving the ball, dipping their shoulders as usual, and then, having feinted to go one way, accelerating rapidly in their less preferred direction. Such visualization practice is best undertaken in conjunction with the physical warm-up routines that precede regular training. Finally, some helpful practical guidelines on the use of imagery in sport are provided by Hale (1998).

Simulation training. The concept of simulation training (Orlick, 1990), also known as "adversity training" (Loehr, 1986), "dress rehearsal" (Schmid &

Peper, 1998), "simulated practice" (Hodge & McKenzie, 1999), and "distraction training" (Maynard, 1998), is based on the assumption that sport performers may become inured against the adverse effects of distractions in competition by practicing systematically in their presence during training. ✕ Notes.

Anecdotal testimonials to the value of this hypothesis are plentiful in sport, both in individual events and in team games. To illustrate the former, Darrell Pace, a two-time Olympic archery champion, reported that, as a novice, he used to practice shooting arrows under noisy and distracting conditions in order to simulate competitive situations: "I shot by railroad tracks, had cars driving by, etc., to practice dealing with distractions. I had to learn to block everything out" (cited in Vealey & Walter, 1994, p. 431). With regard to adversity training for teams, consider how the Australian women's hockey team prepared for the 1988 Olympic Games in Seoul, a tournament that they won by defeating the home team, Korea, in the final. Briefly, the Australians planned for a possible match against Korea by simulating certain aspects of the competitive environment that they expected to encounter. For example, during training, they arranged for crowd noise to be transmitted over a loud-speaker system so that they would become accustomed to the likely behavior of the partisan Korean crowd in the future. In addition, in practice matches, the coach of the team was required to give his half-time instructions against a cacophony of recorded crowd-noise (Miller, 1997). In a similar vein, at the European Championships in England in 1996, Germany, the eventual winner, constructed a special training pitch in Manchester in an effort to replicate the precise dimensions of Wembley—where the final would be held (Lawrenson, 1996). Simulation training in other team-sports has been noted by Singer et al. (1991), who observed that in American football, coaches often "simulate opposing team fans and stadium loud noises during practice to acquaint their players with the potential distracting situations in the subsequent competitive game" (p. 101). Likewise, Schmid and Peper (1998) claimed that many American football coaches turn on water sprinklers during practice matches in preparation for games that are likely to be affected by rain. In Table 2, some examples are offered to illustrate the use of simulation training in soccer.

Unfortunately, despite its intuitive appeal, simulation training has received little or no empirical scrutiny as a concentration technique. However, support for its theoretical advantages may be found in cognitive psychology. For example, research on the "state dependency" of learning shows that information is recalled best "when there is a close match between the conditions in which it was originally learned and the conditions in which the person tries to remember it" (Brewin, 1988, p. 57). The implication of this principle is that by simulating competitive situations in practice, athletes can learn to optimally transfer their training experiences. Also, adversity training can be justified on the grounds that it counteracts the tendency for novel or unexpected factors to distract sports performers in competition. Simulating these factors in training will reduce their subsequent attention-capturing qualities. Finally, simulation training has some physiological plausibility. For example, in order to prepare for the climatic conditions anticipated in the 1986 World Cup in Mexico, members of the Danish national soccer squad trained wearing equipment that progressively lowered the oxygen content of the air that they breathed (Bangsbo, 1994). Taken together, therefore, there are several theoretical grounds to justify the claim that simulation training is a potentially valuable concentration strategy in team sports.

Distraction	Simulation
Crowd noise	Playing prerecorded audiotapes of crowd noise during training sessions to familiarize players with expected stimuli
Gamesmanship/ intimidation	Arranging for teammates to simulate opponents' gamesmanship during practice matches
Fatigue	Alternating normal training sessions with short bouts of high-intensity exercise to induce tiredess
Heat/humidity	Arranging for players to train and play wearing layers of extra clothing to simulate certain climatic effects
Unfavorable refereeing decisions	Designing "modified" games containing deliberately biased umpiring decisions
Pressure	Simulating pressure situations in training (e.g., team losing 1-0 with 5 minutes to go; playing with 10 players against 11)

Table 2. Simulation training in soccer (based on Sellars, 1996)

Now that some theoretical principles and practical techniques encountered in the field of concentration training with team-sport performers have been explored, it is time to sketch some key implications for researchers and practitioners in this field.

New Directions in Research on Concentration Skills Training

At least six potentially significant new directions may be identified for research in the field of concentration skills training. To begin, we need to explore further the question of why even expert athletes appear to be so distractible. In particular, research is required to establish the theoretical mechanisms underlying the "internal" (or self-generated) distractions experienced by these sport performers (see also Hatzigeorgiadis & Biddle, 2000). Until the advent of Wegner's (1994) model of ironic processes, psychologists had largely ignored the effect of people's own thoughts, feelings, and emotions on their attentional processes. Clearly, what is now required is the systematic testing of this model in the field of sport psychology (for some interesting suggestions in this regard, see Janelle, 1999). A second fruitful avenue for further research on concentration in sport concerns the task of exploring "meta-attentional" processes in athletes—or their theories about how their own concentration systems work. This topic is intriguing because most sports performers have developed, out of their competitive experience, informal models of the way in which their minds work. As yet, however, we know very little about the nature, accuracy, and modifiability of these models. Consequently, a number of questions surround them. For example, do sport performers' meta-cognitive models become more sophisticated with increasing athletic expertise? How do these models change as athletes learn to use new concentration techniques? Research is needed to address these questions if only because all attempts at concentration training involve meta-cognitive factors. To explain, athletes cannot learn how to concentrate effectively unless they gain some degree of insight into, and control of, their own mental processes. Third, research is required to evaluate the validity of the various concentration techniques promulgated rather uncritically by some sport psychologists (e.g., Bull et al., 1996; Schmid & Peper, 1998). At present, most of these techniques can be described as plausible but scientifically unproven. Fourth, sport psychologists should explore the relationship between the structure of various athletic activities and their concomitant attentional demands. For example, do untimed games such as golf place demands on the concentration system of performers different from those imposed by timed activities (e.g., soccer)? If so, what theoretical mechanisms could account for such differences? Unless this type of research is undertaken, researchers will not be able to scientifically tailor the components of generic attentional training programs to sport-specific situations. Fifth, what is the best way to measure individual differences in attentional skills? This question was addressed comprehensively by Abernethy et al. (1998). Briefly, these authors reviewed three types of attentional tests: behavioral measures (e.g., "dual-task" tests that assess people's skill in effectively dividing their attention between concurrent actions), psychophysiological indices (see also Hatfield & Hillman, 2001), and cognitive/self-report scales (e.g., the Test of Attentional and Interpersonal Style, TAIS; Nideffer, 1976). Following a review of relevant empirical evidence, they concluded that all three categories of measures should be combined by researchers who wish to measure adequately the multidimensional construct of attention in sport. Unfortunately, as they pointed out, sport psychology researchers in the past tended to select measures of attention more for reasons of brevity and convenience than on grounds of construct validity. For this reason, a welcome addition to attentional measures in sport is a theoretically based scale designed to assess the distractions experienced by athletes in competitive situations (Hatzigeorgiadis & Biddle, 2000). Finally, evaluative research is required to establish the efficacy of attentional skills training programs in sport psychology. In this regard, Ziegler (1995) used a single-case design to demonstrate that two male collegiate soccer players could be trained to shift their attention as required by the demands of various sport-specific tasks. Unfortunately, research suggests that generalized visual-skills training programs are not effective in enhancing soccer performance (Williams, 2000; see also Starkes, Helsen, & Jack, 2001)—a fact that raises serious questions about the validity of using visual search tasks like the "concentration grid" (Schmid & Peper, 1998) as alleged concentration training tools.

Practical Implications for Coaches

Having reviewed relevant theory and research on concentration processes, let us now summarize some practical advice for coaches who are interested in helping team-sport performers to focus optimally (see also Simons, 1999). First, instead of angrily exhorting athletes to "concentrate," coaches should attempt to specify as precisely as possible exactly what performers should focus on in any given situation. As Simons (1999) pointed out, "the bottom line of appropriate focus is for the performer to be clear about what she or he needs to pay attention to and what actions are desired" (p. 101). Second, coaches should try to help athletes to concentrate only on actions that are specific, relevant, and under their own control. The various concentration strategies outlined in this chapter are based on this simple yet powerful principle. Third, it is essential for coaches to try to understand the distractions that afflict their performers in competitive situations. Without such analysis, it is difficult to imagine how typical distractions can be simulated in practice or training. Finally, by helping athletes to develop appropriate plans and routines for "what if" situations in competition, coaches can empower their performers to become self-reliant. Interestingly, in an effort to achieve this objective, one of the first initiatives undertaken by Sven Goran Eriksson after he became manager of the English national soccer team in 2000 was to hire a sport psychologist as a consultant to the players and coaching staff.

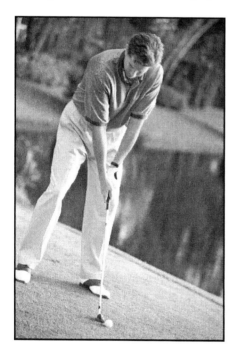

Researchers have yet to discover whether a timed playing period affects an athlete's ability to concentrate.

Summary

Concentration, or the ability to focus mental effort on what is most important in any situation while ignoring distractions, is a vital determinant of athletic success. This principle was illustrated at the beginning of the chapter by describing two errors that resulted from attentional lapses in a top-class soccer match. This example led to an analysis of the nature and importance of concentration in sport. Briefly, we explained that concentration is often likened to a mental spotlight that sport performers shine at things in which they are interested. Using this analogy, we discovered that athletes' concentration is never really "lost," but merely redirected at some target that is irrelevant to the task at hand. This insight led to a distinction between "external" and "internal" distractions in sport. The former consist mainly of environmental factors (e.g., crowd noise, "gamesmanship" by opponents) that divert athletes' attention away from task-relevant concerns. The latter comprise a vast array of self-generated thoughts, feelings, and bodily sensations (e.g., fatigue) that disrupt concentration by narrowing the beam of our mental spotlight and by directing it towards irrelevant factors. Following a brief exploration of some typical distractions encountered in soccer, a set of theoretical principles of concentration that emerge from relevant research findings was specified. Perhaps the most important of these principles is the idea that optimal concentration is achieved when players focus on actions that are specific, relevant, and under their own control. Next, five practical techniques that can be used to improve the concentration skills of soccer players were outlined and illustrated. These techniques included specifying performance goals, using preshot routines, learning arousal-control strategies, using "trigger words" as attentional cues, engaging in mental practice or "visualization," and using simulation training (whereby players train under conditions that mimic anticipated distractions so that they can become accustomed to them when they occur in competitive situations). The chapter concluded with an outline of some potentially fruitful new directions for further research on concentration skills training, as well as a summary of practical advice for coaches who wish to work in this field.

Acknowledgments

I wish to express my sincere gratitude to Ms. Toni Johnson (former administrative assistant) and Mr. Jimmy McDermott (coach, Football Association of Ireland), who helped me in the preparation of this chapter. I also wish to acknowledge some constructive suggestions received from Ronnie Lidor.

References

Abernethy, B. (2001). Attention. In R. N. Singer, H. A. Hausenblas, & C. M. Janelle (Eds.), *Handbook of sport psychology* (2nd ed., pp. 53-85). New York: John Wiley.

Abernethy, B., Summers, J. J., & Ford, S. (1998). Issues in the measurement of attention. In J. L. Duda (Ed.), *Advances in sport and exercise psychology measurement* (pp. 173-193). Morgantown, WV: Fitness Information Technology.

Atkinson, R. C., & Shiffrin, R. M. (1968). Human memory: A proposed system and its control processes. In K. W. Spence & J. T. Spence (Eds.), *The psychology of learning and motivation* (Vol. 2, pp. 89-105). London: Academic Press.

Bangsbo, J. (1994). *Fitness training in football: A scientific approach.* Copenhagen: August Krogh Institute, University of Copenhagen.

Best, G. (1990). *The good, the bad and the bubbly.* London: Pan Books.

Borkovec, T. D., Robinson, E., Pruzinsky, T., & DePree, J. A. (1983). Preliminary exploration of worry: Some characteristics and processes. *Behaviour Research and Therapy, 21,* 9-16.

Brewin, C. R. (1988). *Cognitive foundations of clinical psychology.* Hove, East Sussex: Lawrence Erlbaum.

Bull, S. J., Albinson, J. G., & Shambrook, C. J. (1996). *The mental game plan.* Eastbourne, East Sussex: Sport Dynamics.

Couture, R. T., Jerome, W., & Tihanyi, J. (1999). Can associative and dissociative strategies affect the swimming performance of recreational swimmers? *The Sport Psychologist, 13,* 334-343.

Crews, D. J., & Boutcher, S. H. (1986). Effects of structured preshot behaviours on beginning golf performance. *Perceptual and Motor Skills, 62,* 291-294.

Driskell, J.E., Copper, C., & Moran, A. (1994). Does mental practice enhance performance? *Journal of Applied Psychology, 79,* 481-492.

Dunn, J. G. H. (1999). A theoretical framework for structuring the content of competitive worry in ice hockey. *Journal of Sport and Exercise Psychology, 21,* 259-279.

Easterbrook, J. A. (1959). The effects of emotion on cue utilization and organization of behaviour. *Psychological Review, 66,* 183-201.

Evening Herald. (1999, September 17). *Evening Herald,* p. 38.

Fanning, D. (1999). Cunningham arms himself for battle. *Sunday Independent,* 3 October p. 27.

Fernandez-Duque, D., & Johnson, M. L. (1999). Attention metaphors: How metaphors guide the cognitive psychology of attention. *Cognitive Science, 23,* 83-116.

Fitness - a prerequisite for the enjoyment of soccer at all levels. (2000, January 24). *Evening Herald,* p. 36.

Hale, B. (1998). *Imagery training: A guide for sports coaches and performers.* Headingley, Leeds: The National Coaching Foundation.

Hatfield, B. D., & Hillman, C. H. (2001). The psychophysiology of sport: A mechanistic understanding of the psychology of superior performance. In R. N, Singer, H. A. Hausenblas, & C. M. Janelle (Eds.), *Handbook of Sport Psychology* (2nd ed., pp. 362-388). New York: John Wiley.

Hatzigeorgiadis, A., & Biddle, S. J. H. (2000). Assessing cognitive interference in sport: Development of the thought occurrence questionnaire for sport. *Anxiety, Stress, and Coping, 13,* 65-86.

Hodge, K., & McKenzie, A. (1999). *Thinking rugby.* Auckland, New Zealand: Reed Publishing.

Irish Times (2000, September 2). Reiziger outburst at Keane, p. 1 (Sports Saturday).

Jackson, S. A. (1995). Factors influencing the occurrence of flow state in elite athletes. *Journal of Applied Sport Psychology, 7,* 138-166.

Jackson, R. C., & Baker, J. S. (2001). Routines, rituals, and rugby: Case study of a world class goal kicker. *The Sport Psychologist, 15,* 48-65.

Jackson, S. A., & Csikszentmihalyi, M. (1999). *Flow in sports.* Champaign, IL: Human Kinetics.

Jackson, S. A., & Roberts, G. C. (1992). Positive performance states of athletes: Toward a conceptual understanding of peak performance. *The Sport Psychologist, 6,* 156-171.

Janelle, C. M. (1999). Ironic mental processes in sport: Implications for sport psychologists. *The Sport Psychologist, 13,* 201-220.

Janelle, C. M., Singer, R. N., & Williams, A. M. (1999). External distractions and attentional narrowing: Visual search evidence. *Journal of Sport and Exercise Psychology, 21,* 70-91.

Jones, S. (1995, December 11). Inside the mind of perfection. *The Independent,* pp. 10-11 [Independent Sport].

Lacey, D. (1997, January 23). In search of le panache, *The Irish Times,* p. 5.

Lawrenson, M. (1996, June 27). Attention to detail sees the Germans through. *The Irish Times,* p. 25.

Lewin, K. (1951). *Field theory in social science*. New York: Harper.

Lidor, R., & Singer, R. N. (2002). Preperformance routines in self-paced tasks: Developmental and educational considerations. In R. Lidor & K. Henschen (Eds.), *Psychology of team sports* (pp. 69-98). Morgantown, WV: Fitness Information Technology.

Loehr, J. E. (1986). *Mental toughness training for sports: Achieving athletic excellence*. New York: The Stephen Green Press.

Logie, R. H. (1999). Working memory. *The Psychologist, 12,* 174-178.

Lovejoy, J. (1995, December 3). England's striking success. *The Sunday Times* [sport section], p. 19.

Mallett, C. J., & Hanrahan, S. J. (1997). Race modeling: An effective cognitive strategy for the 100m sprinter? *The Sport Psychologist, 11,* 72-85.

Masters, K. S., & Ogles, B. M. (1998). Associative and dissociative cognitive strategies in exercise and running: 20 years later, what do we know? *The Sport Psychologist, 12,* 253-270.

Maynard, I. (1998). *Improving concentration*. Headingley, Leeds: The National Coaching Foundation.

Miller, B. (1997). *Gold minds: The psychology of winning in sport*. Marlborough, Wiltshire: The Crowood Press.

Moran, A. (1996). *The psychology of concentration in sport performers: A cognitive analysis*. Hove, East Sussex: Psychology Press / Taylor & Francis.

Moran, A. (1998). *The pressure putt* [a golf psychology audiotape]. Aldergrove, Co. Antrim, N. Ireland: Tutorial Services [UK] Ltd.

Moran, A. (2000). Improving sporting abilities: Training concentration skills. In J. Hartley & A. Branthwaite (Eds.), *The applied psychologist* (2nd ed., pp. 92-110). Buckingham: Open University Press.

Nideffer, R. M. (1976). The Test of Attentional and Interpersonal Style. *Journal of Personality and Social Psychology, 34,* 394-404.

O'Neill, C. (2001, May 12). Better late than never - Owen. *The Sunday Tribune* [Sport], p. 3.

Orlick, T. (1990). *In pursuit of excellence*. Champaign, IL: Leisure Press.

Reds boss to hold his fire. (2001, April 20). *Evening Herald*, pp. 94-95.

Reilly, T. (1999, September 5). Just how fit are Gaelic footballers? *The Sunday Tribune*, p. 7.

Reisberg, D. (2001). *Cognition* (2nd ed.). New York: Norton.

Schmid, A., & Peper, E. (1998). Strategies for training concentration. In J. M. Williams (Ed.), *Applied sport psychology: Personal growth to peak performance* (3rd ed., pp. 316-328). Mountain View, CA: Mayfield.

Sellars, C. (1996). *Mental skills: An introduction for sports coaches.* Headingley, Leeds: National Coaching Foundation.

Selvey, M. (1999, March 4). Fowler may be Liverpool's class bully but he is a long way short of a master's degree in the art of sledging. *The Guardian* [Sport], p. 25.

Simon, J. M., & Reeves, J. A. (1985). *The soccer games book.* Champaign, IL: Leisure Press.

Simons, J. (1999). Concentration. In M. A. Thompson, R. A. Vernacchia, & W. E. Moore (Eds.), *Case studies in applied sport psychology: An educational approach* (pp. 89-114). Dubuque, IA: Kendall/Hunt.

Singer, R.N., Cauraugh, J.H., Tennant, L.K., Murphey, M., Chen, D., & Lidor, R. (1991). Attention and distractors: Considerations for enhancing sport performance. *International Journal of Sport Psychology, 22,* 95-114.

Solso, R. (1998). *Cognitive psychology* (5th ed.). Boston: Allyn & Bacon.

Starkes, J. L., Helsen, W., & Jack, R. (2001). Expert performance in sport and dance. In R. N. Singer, H. A. Hausenblas, & C. M. Janelle (Eds.), *Handbook of sport psychology* (2nd ed., pp. 174-201). New York: John Wiley.

Syer, J. (1989). *Team spirit.* London: Simon & Schuster.

Thornley, G. (1993, June 2). Fernandez beats Sabatini in marathon. *The Irish Times,* p. 17.

Townsend, A. (1999, October 15). Ireland's case for the defence. *Evening Herald,* p. 45.

Vealey, R. S., & Walter, S. M. (1994). On target with mental skills: An interview with Darrell Pace. *The Sport Psychologist, 8,* 428-441.

Wegner, D. M. (1994). Ironic processes of mental control. *Psychological Review, 101,* 34-52.

Wegner, D. M., Ansfield, M., & Pilloff, D. (1998). The putt and the pendulum: Ironic effects of the mental control of action. *Psychological Science, 9,* 196-199.

Wegner, D. M., Broome, A., & Blumberg, S. J. (1997). Ironic effects of trying to relax under stress. *Behaviour Research and Therapy, 35,* 11-21.

Wegner, D. M., Eich, E., & Bjork, R. A. (1994). Thought suppression. In D. Druckman & R. A. Bjork (Eds.), *Learning, remembering, believing: Enhancing human performance* (pp. 277-293). Washington, DC: National Academy Press.

Wenzlaff, R. M., & Wegner, D. M. (2000). Thought suppression. *Annual Review of Psychology, 51,* 59-91.

Whitaker, D. (1999). *The spirit of teams.* Marlborough, Wiltshire: The Crowood Press.

White, J. (1999, March 4). Queering the pitch. *The Guardian,* p. 2 (G2).

Williams, M. (2000). Visual performance enhancement in football: Myth or reality? *Insight - The FA Coaches Association Journal, 2,* p. 24.

Ziegler, S. G. (1995). The effects of attentional shift training on the execution of soccer skills: A preliminary investigation. *Journal of Applied Behavioural Analysis, 27,* 545-552.

Zukier, H., & Hagen, J.W. (1978). The development of selective attention under distracting conditions. *Child Development, 49,* 870-873.

CHAPTER 10

Issues for the Sport Psychology Professional in Baseball

Tom Hanson and Ken Ravizza

Abstract

Two consultants share their perspectives and experiences serving as sport psychology professionals in baseball. Topics include the principal objectives of their work (long-term excellent performance, self-adjustment, and consistency); a review of key elements of baseball and baseball culture that affect consultants; the vital role of building relationships, credibility, and trust; and common issues they discuss with players. The role of consultants' authenticity is emphasized, as is the importance of linking the mental game and physical game, "getting" a player, making distinctions, and helping players develop self-control. The authors list common errors in thinking that players make and offer their thoughts on how consultants can get started working in baseball.

Baseball players typically report that 80% or more of their performance is determined by mental and emotional factors. Although some players, particularly younger ones, need to be convinced that their mind plays a critical role in how well they play, most realize that their own thought processes largely determine how well they perform. Coaches are well versed in the technical and strategic aspects of the game, but few possess the knowledge and methods to teach confidence, focus, and consistency directly. As a result, the players' psychological and emotional development is left largely to chance.

Our task as sport psychology professionals is to educate players and coaches on the fundamentals of the mental game and provide a structure of support for them as they develop their abilities to use their thoughts and emotions to their best advantage. Long Beach State Head Coach Dave Snow commented that "incorporating the mental game into my coaching has provided me with a vocabulary to address one of the most important aspects of baseball" (personal communication, September 1996).

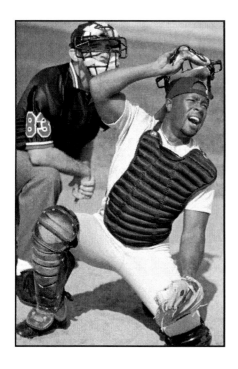

Coaches must consider not only the technical aspects of the game, but also what most players realize—that performance is affected by thoughts and emotions.

In this chapter we share what we have learned as sport psychology professionals working in baseball, including

1. Our principal objectives;
2. The importance of understanding the nature of baseball;
3. The building of relationships, credibility, and trust; and
4. Common issues we address with players.

Objectives of Our Approach

As sport psychology professionals we (a) provide information, (b) teach skills, and (c) support players and coaches in refining and developing their mental approach to the game (Ravizza, 1990). We have three general objectives in our work.

Long-Term Excellent Performance

Our approach is educational, designed to facilitate long-term top performance. Like physical skills, the perspectives and skills we offer players are developed over time. It takes consistent practice over a prolonged period of time for a pitcher to learn to throw a slider, and it takes consistent practice over a prolonged period of time for a player to learn to control his focus. The player's reward for doing the work in both cases is knowing he gave himself his best chance for success.

We take great strides to get players and coaches to understand that we are not "shrinks" to be conferred with only when a player needs to be "fixed." In professional baseball, each team has an employee assistance program that provides counseling services for players and coaches. We refer players to counselors when that is appropriate, but distinguish ourselves as being focused on enhancing performance rather than resolving psychological problems.

Self-Adjustment

Baseball is a game of adjustments, and players need to learn to make adjustments on their own. We want players to develop the ability to recognize when they are not in control of themselves and to have the ability to regain their composure and focus. We want players to be able to realize for themselves when they are too focused on statistics or are not being themselves on the field. The skilled batter makes an adjustment during or between at-bats, whereas the less skilled may give away a game or a whole week's worth of at-bats before making an adjustment.

Consistency, or Making Bad Days Less Bad and Less Frequent

Working on the mental game is not about players being in the "zone" all the time. Often, once a player has developed his mental game, he will find that he is simply more consistent and that the days he plays poorly are not as bad. He begins to report having "good bad days."

The Nature of Baseball

One of the keys to successful consulting in baseball is understanding the nature of the game and the unique challenges it presents. The fundamental elements of top human performance, such as motivation, confidence, focus, and mental preparation, are as critical in baseball as they are in any other performance domain, but it is important to have a firm grasp on the unique combination of factors that make the game so mentally challenging.

The rules of baseball (such as requiring batters to hit a round ball with a round bat, putting nine players out on defense, and forcing pitchers to throw the ball over the plate) are made with the express purpose of making things difficult. The originators of baseball established rules that make it difficult to achieve the results the players want. Part of the enjoyment of the game is overcoming these obstacles.

One of the biggest obstacles for the skilled player is himself—his own thinking and the way he responds internally to the external obstacles the game presents. Our work with the mental game focuses on helping players and coaches overcome the obstacles they put in their own way, including fear, doubt, anxiety, and lack of focus. We help players get out of their own way. The goal is to help the player arm himself with the mind-set and skills he needs to free himself to engage with the external obstacles, with minimal hindrance from himself (Hanson, 1991; Ravizza & Hanson, 1995).

The following section reviews some of the principal aspects of baseball that give rise to the issues most commonly encountered by sport psychology professionals.

Results Are Not Within Players' Control

Success in baseball is usually measured in wins and losses, hits and outs, putouts and errors, but because of the way the game is designed, players fail constantly. Hitting is the most obvious mental challenge: If the batter keeps his failure rate down to 70%, he is a great hitter. Given that professional players play nearly every day, and college players play several days each week, they usually do not have long after a great performance before they fail in the next one. The sentiment is often that a player is only as good as his last performance.

Players often experience frustration because many of the factors that determine their success are outside their control. They can do everything "right" and still fail. The pitcher can watch his best pitch fly over the outfield fence or be called a ball by the umpire. The hitter can hit a ball perfectly and be out before he has a chance to take a step toward first base. A team can be totally focused, play great, but still be beaten by an inferior team because the breaks just went their way. So day after day, month after month, players have to deal with not being able to control whether they achieve the results they want to achieve. Getting players to recognize and accept what they can and cannot control is one of the keys to successfully working in baseball (Dorfman & Kuehl, 1989; Ravizza & Hanson, 1995).

The Players Have Time to Think

Time is another major issue. Players and coaches invest an enormous amount of time in the game. First, baseball players spend many hours at the ballpark. Professional players often get to the field at 2 p.m. for a 7:30 p.m. game, play for 3 hours, then take another hour to shower and clean up before they leave. College players usually spend slightly less time on the field, but still rarely get to the park less than 2 hours before game time. Half the games are on the road, so travel time adds up, and in some pro leagues, players endure 14-hour bus rides.

The routine at the ballpark can become monotonous: Get dressed, stretch out, take batting practice, and wait for the game to start. This cycle is done day after day for six months. Players can easily slip into a "cruise control" mentality and simply put in their time. Players often "go through the motions" of practicing without being mentally and emotionally engaged in what they are doing. As a result, they often lack the intensity and purpose needed to develop their skills and play their best baseball. Enhancing the quality of practice time must be one of the main goals of the mental training program.

No clock is used in baseball, so the game itself takes a long time. The time between pitches can be helpful for a player, but it is often used poorly. Boredom is a major issue. Both before and during the game, the relative lack of action provides ample opportunities for the mind to drift to other interests or concerns. Because of the amount of failure the players experience, it is common for a player to spend much of the time between pitches dwelling on past failures and criticizing himself for a poor performance. He may also spend time between pitches worrying about future pitches. This creates a mind-set that jeopardizes the quality of upcoming performances. Much of the work we do as sport psychology consultants in the mental game focuses primarily on how to best use the time between pitches.

In short, baseball players have an enormous amount of time to think about their performance before, during, and after a game. A player's success in baseball is heavily influenced by what he chooses to focus on during those times.

Baseball Is a Game of Adjustments

Because of the difficulty of the game, the long season of playing every day, and the length and nature of the games, baseball is a game of adjustments. Rarely does a player feel 100% physically or mentally. The long hours and sudden spurts of vigorous activity during the games result in fatigue, soreness, and nagging injuries, so players must constantly adjust to how they feel physically; the challenges of the game (and of life) also force players to constantly adjust to how they feel emotionally.

Baseball is a complex game requiring refined mental and emotional skills, so another challenge is getting to the emotional and psychological state that optimizes performance. Baseball is a marathon consisting of hundreds of short sprints. A high degree of skill is needed to play the game, and the games take hours to play, which suggests that a low level of arousal would generally be most effective; but baseball also requires periodic bursts of high-intensity action, so there are times when a high level of arousal is best (Weinberg & Gould, 1999). Each individual differs as to what arousal level he performs best at, and each position has slightly different demands.

Finally, the game situation changes with each of the approximately 240 pitches thrown. The score, the inning, the weather, the position of the batter in the lineup, where a batter hit the ball the last time up, how the batter looked on the last swing he took, what the batter did against this pitcher two weeks ago, whether the pitcher is getting his breaking ball over for strikes, and the position of runners on base are just some of the variables that must be considered before deciding on a plan for the next pitch. Pitcher Jim Abbott stated that "pitching is like crossing a river, you never can cross the same one twice. The river is always changing like the game is always changing" (personal communication, January 14, 1992).

The ability to think clearly between pitches is critical. If a player's mind is racing from the stress or fear of the situation, he will be unable to make the adjustments the game requires. As Long Beach State Head Coach Dave Snow says, "Working on the mental game is about helping players get where they need to be when they need to be there." This may sound simple, but it is extremely difficult to do in the midst of performance.

Baseball Is an Individual Sport Played in a Team Context

More than most team sports, baseball is individual in nature. The hitter stands alone against the entire opposing team. The third baseman cannot get help on a ball hit sharply down the line. The pitcher is responsible for setting the pace of the game. Add the enormous emphasis placed on statistics in baseball, and there is no hiding. Baseball forces players to "stand naked before the gods" (Metheny, 1969, p. 69).

Future Hall of Famer Wade Boggs said, "This is a team sport made up of nine individuals. No one is going to throw a block for me or set a pick for me or give me an assist when I step into that batter's box to try to help the club" (qtd. in Williamson, 1999a). In other words, as some professional athletes state: "There is no 'I' in the word team, but there is an 'm' and an 'e.'" This is particularly true at the professional level in the minor leagues where the players' focus is to advance their skills and move up to the big leagues. The success of the team is a distant second in importance. Lee Mazzilli, former major leaguer turned manager, says that as a result "baseball can be a lonely, lonely job" (personal communication, March 14, 1999).

One significant difference between the college and pro game is that although the roster of a pro team changes throughout the season, a college team has a set group of players for the whole season. If the college team is going to do well over the course of a full season, the coach needs to develop all the players because each will have to contribute at some point.

Baseball Has a Unique Culture

Like any other sport, baseball has a unique subculture defined by unwritten rules and norms. Acting in accordance with the norms is critical for the sport psychology professional. Below are a few key elements of baseball culture, primarily at the professional level. Keep in mind, though, that the only way to really understand the culture is to be in it.

Two major perspectives operate in the game: "Old School" and "New School." One part of Old School is that baseball is a macho culture. Testosterone abounds. Many players and coaches are reluctant to discuss the mental aspects of the game because in the macho culture this connotes weakness. These players and coaches will tell you they need to work on their mechanics ("It's my swing, I'm pulling my front shoulder") when it's clearly a lack of emotional control hindering their performance. They will tell you that confidence is paramount but not want to talk about it. Denial is prevalent: Players don't want someone else getting in their "dome" (baseball slang for head or mind).

Another implication of this is that players are often reluctant to call the sport psychology consultant even after a strong relationship has been formed and the consultation is free. Players can perceive asking for support as a sign of weakness and believe instead they should work through it on their own.

Coaches and players are often concerned about the problem of players overthinking, and fear a consultant's efforts will result in players thinking too much during their performances. Players consistently report that when they are playing their best they are not thinking about anything, so giving them things to think about will only get in the way. However, they also say they are only in this "not-thinking" mind-set at most 10% of the time. They certainly do not need to do anything differently when they are in that zone, so make it clear that your focus is on what the players do the other 90% of the time.

Superstition is another element of baseball culture. A superstition is something that the player believes brings him good luck or enhances his performance but is not "task relevant." Only in the player's head is wearing the same socks every game connected to pitching well.

If a superstition helps a player to be confident, great. Superstitions are a problem only if a player becomes too dependent on them. A player must still be able to believe he can play a good game even if he can't find his lucky belt or forgets his special necklace at home.

Politics Play a Key Role

All players are not treated the same. In professional baseball minor league players are rated as "prospects" or "nonprospects" by the organization. "Prospects" are given special consideration by the organization and should be given most of your attention. As a consultant, your time is limited and although you'll want to help as many people as you can, you must focus your efforts on the players the organization feels stand the best chance of playing at the Major League level. Identify the prospects and build relationships with them. At the college level, discuss with the head coach the player with whom he would most like to see you spend time, but also realize that nearly all the players will play key roles over the course of the season.

Another issue faced by minor league players is that they often feel they do not know where they stand in the organization, and as a result, they feel frustrated and insecure. Several factors can contribute to this. Organizations often do not want to let the players know their standing because they feel not knowing maximizes motivation, particularly with nonprospects. If players know the organization does not feel they are capable of playing at the major league level, they may quit, leaving the organization without quality players to support the prospects. Also, many players now in the majors were at one time non-prospects who played themselves into prospect status, so an organization is generally slow to rule a player out completely.

Sometimes players' not knowing where they stand is simply poor communication, typical of any large organization. Other times the players simply are not able to hear what they are told about their status, not believing the bad news they hear. This is especially true when a player is sent down or released: He can be so emotionally devastated that he does not hear what is being said. Regardless of their situation, players tend to spend considerable energy wondering what the organization really thinks of them, how other players in the organization at their position are playing, and what their future holds.

The macho culture creates barriers to players expressing these insecurities and ruminations with each other or with the coaching staff, so the issues bounce around inside players' heads and interfere with their performances. A sport psychology professional who can win their trust can be an invaluable resource on this issue by refocusing them back onto factors they can control.

Coaches and Managers Are Critical to Your Success

Minor league coaches and managers almost all have one-year contracts, so they tend to walk on eggshells. There is ample incentive for them to do their jobs well but not stick their necks out for any reason, and the sport psychology professional is sometimes seen as a threat. The implication is that the staff might be slow to support the program, and they might perceive acknowledging your contributions as jeopardizing their position. Get support from the highest possible level. If it's clear that the top person in the organization supports the program, the incentive is there for the staff to support you. Support from the staff is vital to a mental game program. With strong support the players can benefit greatly from the program. With weak support you will struggle to make a difference with the players.

Be constantly aware of territoriality issues. Clearly define the mental game as the focus of your work. Don't coach mechanics—focus on players' thoughts and feelings. This is challenging because the game does not divide neatly into the mental game and the physical game. In fact, one of the keys to being effective is helping players integrate mental skills into the physical performance of the game. Keep in mind, however, that in most cases talking mechanics with players will jeopardize your job.

You must collaborate with the coaches to get the job done because they are with the players every day and can support the consultant's work. Keep the staff well informed on what you are doing, but also make sure the coaches are aware of the need for confidentiality in conversations with players—you can't afford to be seen as a "spy" for management.

Coaches work long and hard for very little money to develop players. Avoid media acknowledgment for your work with a player who has performed well. Sport psychology makes for a sexy story, but a story about you creates the risk of fostering resentment from a coach who works with the player every day and is more likely responsible for the player's improvement. Some consultants request that players not mention the work they've done to avoid such possibilities.

In summary, we have addressed some of the key elements of the nature of baseball that influence your effectiveness as a sport psychology professional. These will provide some insight for which issues to address and which to avoid as you enter the baseball culture.

Relationships, Credibility, and Trust

Relationships are another key to success (Ravizza, 1988). Everything is made easier or more difficult by the quality of the relationships you create. Your ability to establish rapport, be seen as credible, and be trusted determines the impact you have. If no one listens to you, it doesn't matter what you know. To be effective as a sport psychology professional in baseball, you must be perceived as credible and trustworthy (Dorfman, 1990; Ravizza, 1990; Smith & Johnson, 1990).

The key to being able to develop good relationships with others is to first develop a solid relationship with yourself. You must be authentic. Even the most die-hard, Old School coaches will be open to you and to sport psychology if what you say resonates with their experience. Even the rawest of rookies can see through a consultant trying to be something he or she is not. How you are must be congruent with what you are talking about. Nonverbal communication can be much more effective than verbal communication, so what you know is less important than how you are perceived by players and coaches.

How do you become authentic? The same way players get good—they do the work. Practice and develop the skills you talk about. Learn about yourself by paying attention to what you think and do, working with a counselor, keeping a journal, or participating in training sessions or workshops. Learn baseball by playing it, being around it, and by talking with players and coaches.

We find our best, most helpful stories come from our own experiences. Visualize. Use a routine. Compete. Play the game. Join a softball or adult baseball team and see what goes through your head after you make an error. You can learn a lot by talking with athletes and coaches, and their stories will become an important resource as they complement your direct experience.

To be as effective as you can be, the principles you share with a player must be a part of you; they cannot just be concepts that you've read or heard someone talk about. You don't need to have faced Major League pitching to help a Major League batter, but you do need to have some comparable experience of applying the idea you are discussing with the player. After working with the Anaheim Angels for five years, Ravizza was told that the Major League club no longer wanted his services. The feelings that came with being "sent down" to the minor leagues gave him a new level of compassion for what the players experience when they are given bad news.

Know why you are there. Are you committed to helping people—and baseball is where you want to express this commitment—or are you simply drawn by the allure of working with elite athletes? Sometimes people go into helping professions to avoid dealing with their own personal issues. Focusing on helping others keeps the attention off themselves. Part of doing the work of being authentic is distinguishing why you want to do this work in the first place.

One suggestion is to adopt a mentor or coach to aid your ongoing development. Anyone who is committed to being his or her best has a coach. You are asking players to adopt you as a coach for their mental and emotional development, so it stands to reason that you too would work with a coach. How can you expect a player to give up his resistance to working with a consultant if you aren't willing to be vulnerable enough to be coached by someone else?

Listening is the most important consulting skill. It is a skill you develop with practice when you are committed to helping someone. Again the key issue is knowing yourself and living the skills and perspectives you are teaching. You can't hear what a player is really saying when your own head is awash with fears and self-doubts.

Structure your work in ways that are consistent with who you are and with your experience. Hanson, for example, has coached baseball for 15 years, and it greatly enhances his credibility to be in uniform, throw batting practice, and shag fly balls. Ravizza has worked in professional baseball for 15 years but does not have baseball experience as a player or coach and, like most consultants, does not wear a uniform. The baseball culture is ruthless and will eat up someone who is being inauthentic.

Another way to gain credibility is to publish books and articles. In our society, being an author means being an expert. You gain credibility when people see that you know what you are talking about. Finally, you will be doing your job if you keep the interest of the player foremost in mind.

"Getting" a Player

Coaches and managers talk of the importance of "getting" a player. "Getting" a player means getting his attention and respect so you can help him develop. Until you "get" a player, your ability to influence him is limited.

The fundamental element is caring. When a player knows you really care about him as a person, the opening is created for you to help him improve. Although our approach is educational and not just focused on problem solving, we often have to wait for a "teachable moment"—usually when a player is struggling—before he is willing to talk and listen. When the player knows we care about him as a person, those teachable moments come more often.

There is no set way to get a player; each manager, coach, and consultant must do it in a way consistent with his or her own personal style. Fundamentals of getting a player, however, include establishing honest, direct, and fair communication and demonstrating a solid knowledge of the game, a strong work ethic, integrity, honesty, loyalty, patience, compassion, consistency, and organization.

So the principal issue for the sport psychology professional is building relationships and gaining credibility and trust with the person bringing you in, the athletes, and the coaches. Authenticity and caring are the key elements. The degree to which you bring yourself and your own experiences to the situation rather than just knowledge you have read in books determines much of your success. If you tell the players to trust themselves while performing, you must be able to do the same. Players' trust in you will be largely determined by the degree to which they sense your trust in yourself.

Getting Started

The best way to learn is to talk with players and coaches. There is no substitute for hearing things straight from players. Fortunately there is a simple way to do this. Ask managers and coaches if you can interview their players for a project you are doing on confidence or mental preparation. Interviewing players gives you stories and firsthand knowledge of the key issues players face, and it also demonstrates that you want to learn from the player. In addition, you also quickly discover that although the athletes have developed special skills in baseball, they still have the trials and tribulations that all humans face.

Players are often reluctant to ask for help with the mental game. Begin a conversation by asking the player to help you. Tell the player you are looking to learn more about confidence in baseball, and you want his perspective. As you progress, players will talk about their confidence; ask what helps their confidence and what hurts it. Ask questions, and players will learn from their own answers, making useful new distinctions about themselves and what they need to do to be their best. As the energy of the conversation begins to wind down, thank them and tell them they have been a big help.

Be authentic. Really want to learn from them. If you are manipulative, they will recognize it. Using this inquiry approach allows players to keep their ego intact and allows you to learn and make a contribution to the player. Again, players are often reluctant to start a conversation, but are generally glad afterwards when you do.

Making Distinctions

People often see sport psychology work solely as teaching mental skills, such as visualization, routines, relaxation, self-talk, focus, breathing, and goal setting. Although these are an important part of our work, examining the way a player is viewing his performance is also a major emphasis.

One of our goals is to have a conversation that alters the way a player is looking at his situation in such a way that it gives him greater freedom to perform to his highest ability. For example, say a pitcher throws great in the bullpen but poorly in a game. Rather than simply teaching the player a routine and relaxation skills, enter into a conversation with him to distinguish what the underlying belief is that has him tense up during the game. What does it mean to him to succeed? What does it mean to fail? What beliefs are giving rise to his fear? It isn't the situation itself that is causing the stress; it's how the player is viewing his situation. Try to distinguish the source of the issue rather than simply treat the symptom.

Here is where rapport-building skills, listening skills, and experience are important. Hear the player's issue, distinguish with him how his current perspective is limiting him, and illustrate your point with a story of another athlete who fell into a similar mental trap (be sure the story is anonymous unless you know the player in the story agrees with your sharing it).

Don't put pressure on yourself to come up with THE brilliant answer. Give a player space to talk and ask him some basic questions, and the player will distinguish something useful for himself. Actually, it's usually best to let a player talk through his situation and come to his own conclusion rather than to lecture him. Simply telling a player to trust himself is not as likely to make a difference for him as his deducing it for himself in a conversation will. This process also helps the player learn to learn from himself.

Keep in mind that the distinction made is almost always the player's remembering something he used to do rather than your teaching him something new. Some of the more common distinctions we see include

1. He has forgotten that baseball is difficult and acts as if it were easy (i.e., becomes overly upset when he makes an out).
2. He has forgotten why he plays baseball in the first place.
3. He began playing baseball because he loved it and now he has made it a job.
4. He used to play baseball, and now it has become work.
5. He has forgotten that he is playing against the best players in the world.
6. He is totally focused on outcomes and statistics instead of the process of playing the game (for example, he is trying to get hits instead of hitting the ball hard).
7. He is focused on what others (front office, manager, family) are thinking of him rather than on being himself.
8. He is trying to play outside of his abilities (a small player trying to hit home runs, a ground-ball pitcher trying to strike guys out).
9. He has tied his self-esteem to his performance (he is a good person when he plays well, a bad person when he does poorly).

Occasionally you will have a conversation where a player has an "Aha!" experience and a significant shift in how he is performing, but more often it is a nondramatic, gradual process. Be patient. Don't try to force some brilliant insight. Your commitment to helping the player is more important than being brilliant.

The next step is to devise a plan to put this new approach into action. If the player's behavior does not change, his performance does not change. Agree to some type of practice that the player is going to adopt. Examples include increasing emotional intensity during batting practice, using a pre-at-bat routine, developing a plan to release negative emotions on the field, and keeping a journal.

Let subsequent conversations focus on whether the player is following the plan he agreed to and what he is observing as a result of the practice. In fact, don't even allow the player to talk to you about his game results (how many hits he got, how many runs he gave up) in order to reinforce the importance of process over results.

Link the Mental Game and the Physical Game

Regardless of the issue you are discussing, if players and coaches do not see the practical application of it, you have no chance of gaining their respect, so it is important to link the "mental game" to the physical game. Make this link by discussing and demonstrating what the player is thinking at specific moments in the game, tying the thoughts to physical movements. For examples of how to do this, see Heads-up Baseball: Playing the Game One Pitch at a Time (Ravizza & Hanson, 1995).

Actually, the distinction between the mental game and physical game is an artificial one, made up through language so we can talk about it more easily. The distinction serves the sport psychology professional because it gives him or her a niche, a place to say, "I work in the mental game." Although there are aspects that seem more mental and others that seem more physical, there are not a mental game and a physical game—it's all baseball.

Make the distinction between mental skills and game strategy. Coaches sometimes think "mental game" only means which pitch to throw when, whether or not to steal a base, or what bunt coverage to run. Mental skills help a player think clearly to make the most effective strategic choice. We do not coach players on which game strategy choice is best.

Integrate the sport psychology knowledge with what the players are doing physically without crossing into coaching mechanics. That's part of the "dance" the sport psychology professional has to do all the time. The better rapport and communication you have with the coaching staff, the less likely you are to have trouble in this area.

Even the term mental game is inadequate because it misses the emotional aspects of performance. An athlete can be mentally focused on the right things but be washed out of his performance state by his own emotional response to a pressure situation (Botterill, Patrick, & Sawatzky, 1996). Thus an athlete has to be emotionally as well as mentally prepared. We're using "mental game" in this chapter because it is established in the baseball culture.

Common Player Issues

Below is a brief discussion of what we feel are the key issues players face in baseball. For more detailed descriptions of these ideas, see Ravizza and Hanson (1995). Another excellent resource is *The Mental Game of Baseball* by Dorfman and Kuehl (1989).

The combination of the nature of baseball and the nature of human beings results in many common mental-game issues. The most frequent of these include players'

1. Focusing on things outside their control (which includes getting caught up in statistics, focusing on results rather than process, and spending time and energy worrying about what moves the general manager or head coach is going to make),
2. Not playing one pitch at a time—carrying previous pitches and at-bats into their present performance,
3. Not having a plan or purpose for each pitch,
4. Not trusting their own ability,
5. Losing connection with why they play the game,
6. Getting into slumps,
7. Overfocusing on mechanics,
8. Trying to be perfect, and
9. Personalizing their performance (linking how they are performing with how they feel about themselves as people).

The goal is for the player to consistently be himself, fully focused and fully trusting himself on each pitch. The only aspect of the game the player can control is himself, so his knowledge of himself is paramount and is the foundation for all mental-game issues. We will also discuss self-control and confidence. Consistency is a thread that runs throughout our work because of the number and frequency of the games played. Any player can be great for a day. The ones who rise to the top play well consistently.

Self-Knowledge

The fundamental challenge for the player is to know himself. Long-time major league pitching coach Billy Connors says, "I want a pitcher to know himself so he can go out there on the mound and be himself" (personal communication, March 1999).

"Knowing yourself" as a baseball player includes knowing why you play baseball, what type of player you are, what thoughts and actions lead to your best performances, what your strengths and weaknesses are, and what your goals are. Self-knowledge is the foundation for other key elements of the mental game, and it includes confidence, focus, mental preparation and regrouping, all of which enable a player to consistently play to the best of his ability.

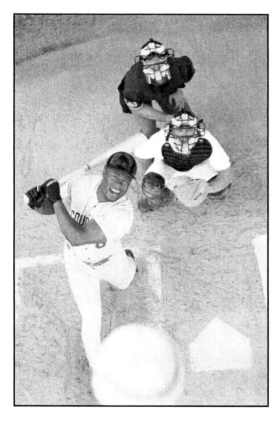

What both players and coaches must realize is that the mental game is a part of, not separate from, the physical game.

Hall-of-Famer Nolan Ryan attributes much of his success to the fact that he constantly studied himself. He knew the nuances of his mechanics, what his workouts needed to be, what he should eat, when he should eat, how much rest he needed, and how he needed to focus during a game. "I paid attention to my body," he said (personal communication, February 1999). Ryan clearly considered his performance a 24-hour-per-day business. All of the choices he made about how to spend his time came from making observations about himself. He continually asked himself: "What do I need to do to be the best player I can be?" His goal was to be consistent, and his incredible record stemmed from his knowledge of what led to his best performances (personal communication, February 1999).

Mark McGwire attributes his success during the past few years to the work he has done getting to know himself as a person. When asked why a few years ago he said he did not like what he saw when he looked in the mirror, McGwire responded:

> I didn't know who I was. I am so firm that you have to be grounded on this earth to be successful. I was floating, I didn't have my feet on the ground. I didn't know who I was, I didn't know what I liked. I went and searched out to get help, which a lot of people shy away from because if they go to see a psychologist, they think there is something wrong with them. Well, I guarantee there is something wrong with everybody on this earth. (Williamson, 1999b)

A principal role of a sport psychology professional is to help players know themselves better. The better a player knows himself, the better choices he is able to make regarding how to spend his time and energy, enabling him to make the most of his ability. Such self-knowledge also helps guard against basing his self-esteem on his performance.

Freedom and Responsibility of Choice

One of the first things a player needs to know about himself is that he has the freedom to determine his perspective on what happens to him. As a human being he has the ability to choose his thoughts and actions, and the thoughts and actions he takes determine his performance. One of the cornerstones of our approach is "You can't control what happens to you, but you can control your response to it." This is good news for the player: Given his physical limitations, he can choose to be the player he wants to be.

The flip side to that freedom is that his thoughts and actions are his responsibility. If he is free to choose his thoughts and actions regardless of his situation, he owes it to his team and himself to think the most performance-enhancing thoughts he possibly can. Going into a depressed, slumping mindset is a selfish act because it hurts the team's chance of winning.

A player does not have to lose confidence after a strikeout. Reggie Jackson said late in his career that he could become more confident after striking out because he now knew how the pitcher would try to get him out. Helping a player understand that he has free will is a first step in enhancing his mental game.

What Are You Doing When You're Playing Great?

A good place to start a conversation with any player is asking him about what he is doing, thinking, and feeling when he is playing his best. Get him to recall a specific game or series when he was in the "zone" or "hot," and ask him questions that make him examine what contributed to this performance. How did he prepare for the game? What did he spend his time thinking about before the game? During the game? What did he focus on? How did he feel while performing? Then use this information to create a preperformance routine (see chapter 4, which focuses on preperformance routines in sport; Ravizza, 1977).

A routine is a set series of mental actions intended to create an "internal climate" that gives players their best chance for success. Adherence to a routine does not guarantee peak performance, but it does set the stage for such a performance to happen. Players seem to understand that having a routine is analogous to going to sleep at night. Just as you can't will yourself into the "zone," you can't will yourself to sleep. You can, though, set the stage for sleep to happen. You go to the bathroom, brush your teeth, change your clothes, get into bed, turn out the light, put your head on the pillow, and close your eyes. This does not guarantee a good night's sleep, but it does make such an outcome more likely.

A preperformance routine does the same thing. What are the steps a player takes that lead to his best performances? What does a hitter do in batting practice, on the bench, on deck and at the plate when he is hitting great? What does a relief pitcher do and think during batting practice, during the first few innings of the game, during his warm-up after he's told to get ready to come in, during his warm-up pitches once he comes into the game, and before each pitch?

The player's preperformance routine is based on his knowledge of himself, of the actions and thoughts he needs to take to give himself his best chance of playing well. It is his recipe for consistent, top-level performance.

Why Do You Play?

Another fundamental question a player should answer for himself is why he plays the game. Ask a player why he plays baseball, and he's likely to say,

"Because I love it." Ask what he loves about it, and he'll likely say, "The competition." You may hear many different answers, but ultimately baseball players play because it provides them with an opportunity to experience feelings they enjoy feeling.

Players who are not performing well usually have lost connection with why they play the game. They once played for the experience of fun, enjoyment, love, passion, and intensity, but now they are experiencing boredom, frustration, anger, or resignation. Their reason for playing needs to be kept center stage to help pull, push, or guide them through the long hours and disappointments of baseball. One former teammate of Roger Clemens said, "You'd never know he was making nine million dollars, he trains and practices and competes so intensely." Clemens does not lose sight of why he plays the game.

Distinguish the feelings a player loves to have while playing the game—at the plate, during his pitching delivery, anticipating the ground ball—and encourage him to learn how to feel these feelings consistently. Pitchers will talk about feeling "free," "fluid," "easy," "natural," "smooth," "powerful," and "rhythm" during their motions. Nonpitchers will say they feel "loose," "relaxed," "cocky," and "confident" to describe how they feel at the plate or on defense.

Ask "If you were committed to feeling 'free, fluid, and easy' throughout the game tonight, how would you do it? What actions and thoughts would you need to take now, during pregame, and during the game that would have you feel that way?" Then the player is to choose to take those actions regardless of his circumstances. He will not be able to create the wonderful feelings he loves to have every day, and he must know he can play very well without feeling very well. Knowing the feeling he wants gives him a clear target to shoot for, adding consistency to his performance (Newburg, 1999).

What Type of Player Are You?

Another key to a player's knowing himself is knowing the type of player he is. Coaches often tell a player to "stay within yourself." What does that mean? In order to stay within himself, a player has to have an accurate assessment of his capabilities and limits. One way to help a player distinguish the type of player he is is to ask him who he thinks is someone else in the Major Leagues who has essentially the same "tools" (ability to run, throw, hit, hit with power, and play defense). His response gives you and the coaching staff an understanding of how well the player understands his abilities.

What Is Your Best Approach?

Many of the obstacles players have to overcome stem from a lack of knowledge about who they are as players and what approach they take to the game when they are playing well. Batting slumps, for example, are often caused by a player's getting away from the approach to hitting that works best for him. Most hitters hit best when they try to hit the ball hard up the middle, but something will happen, such as pulling a ball for a home run, that gets the player trying to pull the ball for more home runs. He is then out in front of pitches, commits himself too soon, and takes long, tense swings with his front shoulder pulling off the ball. This leads to a lot of strikeouts and weak groundouts. After struggling for a while, he will be coached to keep his front shoulder in. This may make things worse because his focus is on his shoulder instead of the ball. Players and coaches often look for a mechanical solution when the problem is in the mental approach.

Eventually the player gets a bloop base hit or a two-strike opposite-field line drive, and he gets the feeling back that he can hit—he feels like his old self. He is now more relaxed, not trying as hard, and focusing on hitting the ball up the middle.

The better a player knows himself and what he does when he is playing well, the less frequently he will stray from his best thinking and the shorter and less severe his slumps will be. The player who pays attention to himself has the best chance to play consistently near his best.

Again, the basic plan is simple:

1. Distinguish the factors that lead to the player's best performances.
2. Establish a structure such as a preperformance routine that will remind him to take those actions before each performance.

Self-Control

Once a player has a sense of what thoughts and actions result in his best performance, the key is to develop the ability to have these thoughts and perform these actions consistently. You may help a player make a distinction, obtain an insight, or develop a routine that enhances his performance in the short run, but if he does not practice it, he will quickly lose it. The player is always free to choose his thoughts and perspective, but unless he chooses them consistently enough to form a new habit, he will almost immediately revert to his more familiar ways of thinking. Mental skills are developed just like physical skills—through practice.

Doing the work of developing the mental game can be compared to doing reps in the weight room or practicing a martial art in that it takes time and effort. It is not a linear process: The player will progress, hit plateaus, and have setbacks. Long-term, consistent top performances result from the consistent application of a strategy. A player will often try something for a short time, and even though he may say it helps him, he will forget about it before long.

The role of the consultant is to provide inspiration, education, and feedback to support the player in developing his mental game. Often this means calling players and initiating conversations and giving players assignments to do between meetings. Two basic skills players can develop to help them better "control" themselves are breathing and visualization. Remind the players: Self-control leads to body control, which leads to ball (or bat) control (Ravizza & Hanson, 1995).

Breathing. Players consistently report that taking a deep breath between pitches is one of the most helpful ideas they hear from us. A full breath (into the belly if possible) helps a player get "centered" and gain control of himself. The breath slows things down for the player, helps him think clearly, and relaxes muscles that have been tensed during the course of the previous pitch.

Visualization and focus. Hank Aaron said his ability to focus is what enabled him to be so incredibly consistent and to put up astronomical career statistics including 755 home runs and 2,297 RBIs. He said visualization was the key to his focus and that it was not something he was born with but rather a skill he developed through years of practice. He visualized facing the pitcher throwing against him all through the day of the game and before each at-bat to prepare himself mentally to lock in his focus (Hanson, 1991).

Bert Blyleven, 273-game winner, says "Visualization is concentration" (Ravizza & Hanson, 1995, p. 57). Seeing in his mind's eye the last 2-3 feet of each pitch just before starting his windup was key to his being focused on one pitch at a time.

Developing these skills enables a player to alter the way he feels and to gain control of himself. Just as important, these skills help a player perform well when he does not feel confident or maybe does not even feel like playing. This can happen often during a season of over 100 games. A player with a strong mental game acts consistently with his commitment to being the player he wants to be rather than simply playing according to how he feels at a given moment.

Confidence

Most players usually say 80% or more of their game is determined by their confidence. They also generally report that the most powerful determinant of their confidence is the results they are producing. Because the results they are producing (getting hits, getting batters out) are outside their control, that means their confidence is outside their control. Nearly everything we do with the players is ultimately intended to enable them to take greater control of their own confidence level.

Players know what they need to do to be confident, but either they are not aware that they know or for some reason they choose not to do it. When asked, players will typically mention that off-the-field actions that can help them be more confident include eating a healthy diet, getting quality rest, using weight training, conditioning, visualizing playing well, and being on top of money issues and also the status of their relationships with their girlfriend, wife, parents, and friends.

Pregame actions that build confidence can include doing drill work, working out, executing well at the plate during batting practice, intently taking balls off the bat during batting practice, and doing "homework" on the opposing hitters or pitcher.

During the game, players report studying the opponent, visualizing successful performances, using preperformance routines, taking deep breaths, and talking with teammates, all of which can help them feel more confident.

After the game a player can help his confidence by reviewing what happened in the game he just played and taking note of what he learned. Some committed players will keep a journal of what they observed about themselves during a game, which in turn greatly facilitates learning. Again, although the distinctions we provide and skills that players develop can help them feel more confident, they also help a player to play well even when he is not confident. Players often make the mistake of thinking good players never lose their belief in themselves. A few days before being inducted to the Hall of Fame, George Brett said, "I was scared to death every time I put on that uniform" (Williamson, 1999a). The key is to have the desire to succeed be greater than the fear (Newburg, 1999).

Other Issues

Players are faced with many other issues than those we have described in this chapter, including planning quality practices, developing mental preparation, breaking out of slumps, dealing with the long season, and establishing relationships with teammates. Helping a player with any of these issues comes back to helping a player get to know himself.

"How should I prepare for a game?" "What should I be focused on at the plate?" "What is the best way for me to pull myself together when I 'lose it' in the middle of an inning?" Although we have noticed recurring themes in different players, the "best" answer to these questions varies with the individual.

The consultant brings his or her past experience with what has worked for other people to each issue, but the objective is to get the player to understand that there is no one "best" solution that works for all players. Help the player determine what works best for him and then develop his ability to use that strategy consistently.

Conclusion

This chapter reviewed the basic issues involved in doing sport psychology work with professional and college baseball teams. Our intent was to help sport psychology professionals and college and professional coaches more effectively enhance the performance of players. We have outlined the principal issues we face when performing sport psychology work in baseball. Most of the observations stemmed from our experiences in professional baseball, but the key issues faced are common to players and coaches at all levels.

As "New School" people gain greater control, baseball is gradually becoming more receptive to sport psychology professionals. The greatest barrier to more people working in the game is the lack of sport psychology professionals possessing the qualities needed to be effective. We hope this chapter will assist consultants in their efforts to be of service to baseball players and coaches.

References

Botterill, C., Patrick, T., & Sawatzky, M. (1996). *Human potential: Perspective, passion, preparation.* Winnipeg, Canada: Lifeskills.

Dorfman, H. (1990). Reflections on providing personal and performance enhancement consulting services in professional baseball. *The Sport Psychologist, 4,* 341-346.

Dorfman, H., & Kuehl, K. (1989). *The mental game of baseball.* South Bend, IN: Diamond Communications.

Hanson, T. (1991). Sport psychology: The mental game. In J. Kendall (Ed.), *Science of coaching baseball* (pp. 25-47). Champaign, IL: Human Kinetics.

Metheny, E. (1969). *Movement and meaning.* New York: McGraw-Hill.

Newburg, D. (1999). *The ultimate competition: Making desire greater than fear.* Unpublished manuscript.

Ravizza, K. (1977). Peak experiences in sport. *The Journal of Humanistic Psychology, 17,* 35-40.

Ravizza, K. (1988). Gaining entry with athletic personnel for season-long consulting. *The Sport Psychologist, 2,* 243-254.

Ravizza, K. (1990). Sportpsych consultation issues in professional baseball. *The Sport Psychologist, 4,* 330-340.

Ravizza, K., & Hanson, T. (1995). *Heads-up baseball: Playing the game one pitch at a time.* Indianapolis: Masters Press.

Smith, R., & Johnson, J. (1990). An organizational empowerment approach to consultation in professional baseball. *The Sport Psychologist, 4,* 347-357.

Weinberg, R. S., & Gould, D. (1999). *Foundations of sport and exercise psychology* (2nd ed.). Champaign, IL: Human Kinetics.

Williamson, N. (News Director). (1999a, July 23). *Sportscenter.* Bristol, CT: ESPN.

Williamson, N. (News Director). (1999b, June 20). *Upclose.* Bristol, CT: ESPN.

CHAPTER 11

The U. S. Women's Olympic Gold Medal Ice Hockey Team: Optimal Use of Sport Psychology for Developing Confidence

Peter Haberl and Leonard Zaichkowsky

Abstract

This chapter is likely different from the many other contributions in this book. Rather than discuss the myriad of skills and techniques we have used in our collective work, we chose to deal with one team and primarily one sport psychology concept. The team is the 1998 gold-medal-winning U.S. women's ice hockey team and the concept is "confidence" (both individual and team). What follows is essentially a story—a story of how a sport psychology consultant worked with USA hockey, the coaching staff, and team members to help the team succeed in Nagano, Japan. Unlike most consulting sport psychologists, this consultant was given permission to collect qualitative and quantitative research data over the period he worked with the team. As such, much of what is said in this chapter comes as data from the players and coaching staff. We begin with how entry was made to become the consulting sport psychologist. This is followed by a brief history of the U.S. Olympic women's hockey team in international competition. We then discuss the concept of individual and team confidence, its importance, sources, barriers, and methods used for fostering confidence in this particular Olympic team. So after providing relevant background information, the focus of this chapter is on the intervention steps taken to develop confidence, supported by player quotes, rather than a presentation of the actual data, which would go beyond the scope of this chapter.

In the fall of 1996, one of the authors was invited to spend one week at a training camp in Lake Placid with the Women's National Ice Hockey team. For all practical purposes, this was a tryout for the sport psychology consultant, to see if the team would respond favorably to sport psychology and the style of the consultant. This unofficial tryout followed the submission of a written proposal to the coaching staff and an extensive lobbying effort to provide comprehensive sport psychology services to the team in preparation for the 1998 Olympic Games. Three months earlier, USA Hockey had announced a new full-time coach, Ben Smith, for the women's national team in preparation for the Nagano Olympics. The 1998 Olympics would be the first time that women's hockey would participate as a full medal sport. It was to be the coming of age of a sport whose roots date back 100 years (McFarlane, 1994).

This initial tryout proved to be successful, at least from the point of continuation, as the consultant was invited to the next training camp. Eventually, over the next two years he spent more and more time with the team, on and off the ice, accompanying them on most of their road trips, to the World Championships in 1997, and eventually joining the team in Nagano at the Olympic Games.

Team History

In 1997 at the World Championships, the team lost the gold medal game in overtime 4-3 to their Canadian hosts in Kitchener, Ontario. This loss was the fourth consecutive defeat for the U. S. team in World Championship finals to the Canadians and set the stage for the upcoming Olympic Games the following year. Clearly, Team Canada was the gold medal favorite. Team USA was considered the underdog, an underdog that had carried the label of having a tendency to choke in big games when "the money" was on the line.

Being considered the underdog did not deter the U. S. team from setting the gold medal as their goal at the Olympics, as the following quote by one of the players on the Olympic team indicates:

> . . . obviously our goal going into the Olympics was gold. I don't think we ever looked at silver, we never thought of silver, but as far as the Canadians being number one, in a way it took pressure off us, they had never lost, they were going to lose at some point, and we were so hungry . . .

For many athletes, the Olympics represent the pinnacle of their career. It is a high point that comes around only every four years, which makes it different from all other competitions, as does the increased pressure, often due to heightened attention from the media as well as from friends and family (Gould et al., 1998). Performing to one's potential at such a pressure-filled event and reaching outcome goals, such as winning the gold medal, is no easy feat. In a recent study of successful and less successful athletes at the 1996 Olympics, Gould and associates (1998) reached the conclusion that achieving peak performance at the Olympics requires the complex interplay of many factors, and one of these factors is mental preparation. Gould et al.'s (1998) study indicated that successful teams and athletes had mentally prepared themselves for the Olympics.

The head coach of Team USA, Ben Smith, having had previous experience coaching at Olympic Games, was very much aware of the importance of mental and emotional preparation in order to compete successfully at this level. Therefore, he was keen on integrating this aspect into his overall preparation of the hockey team for the Olympics. Obviously, mental and emotional preparation itself is a multifaceted process, consisting of components such as learning cognitive strategies for offense and defense, developing commitment to training, preparing for distractions, learning to manage stress and avoid burnout, managing competitive emotions, building concentration and confidence, and fostering team cohesion.

The Importance of Confidence

All of the above mental skills and techniques were addressed as part of the psychological preparation for the Olympic Games. However, due to space constraints and the relative importance of confidence, this chapter will focus on the efforts to help nurture confidence in the Olympic team. The interested reader will find a detailed presentation and discussion of the intervention techniques on the Olympic team in Haberl's (2000) study. Obviously, confidence is an important issue for a team that had lost four times in the deciding gold medal game at various World Championships. Confidence is generally considered one of the most important mental skills for elite athletes to have (Hardy, Jones, & Gould, 1996). Confident athletes are more likely to set challenging goals, are persistent in the pursuit of these goals even in the face of setbacks, and expend more energy in pursuing these goals (Bandura, 1986). Furthermore, it is easier for confident athletes to stay focused on the task at hand, and they experience more positive emotions that often manifest themselves in playing to win, rather than to lose (Weinberg & Gould, 1999). For example, confidence discriminates between successful and less successful gymnasts during Olympic trials (Mahoney & Avener, 1977) and Big Ten wrestlers (Gould, Weiss, & Weinberg, 1981). High self-confidence is one of those psychological attributes associated with peak performance (Williams & Krane, 1998), and although Olympic wrestlers, prior to their best perform-ance, experienced positive expectancies (Gould, Eklund, & S. A. Jackson, 1992a, 1992b), being confident at the Olympics is not easy. In their study of Atlanta Olympians, Gould et al. (1998) reached the conclusion that even in normally confident athletes, confidence can be very fragile at the Olympics.

Confidence plays an important role in the individual athlete's perform-ance, and it also plays an important role for the whole team. Team confidence, or collective efficacy as it is generally termed in the research literature, has been less extensively researched in comparison to individual confidence. According to Bandura (1986), collective efficacy also mediates the behavior of teams, as it "will influence what people choose to do as a group, and how much effort they put into it, and their staying power when group efforts fail to produce results" (p. 449). Feltz and Bandura (1989) suggested that both team and individual confidence should be developed and furthermore that role clarity, role acceptance, and performance are expected to be related to team confidence. For Bandura (1986), collective efficacy is rooted in self-effi-cacy, but whereas strong collective efficacy can raise weak self-efficacy, low collective efficacy does not necessarily undermine strong self-efficacy. This argument further highlights the importance of developing confidence on a group level as well as on an individual level, because it is such a crucial ingre-dient of optimal performance.

Sources of Confidence

This brief review of the literature details the importance of confidence for successful Olympic performance. Furthermore, in order to achieve optimal performance at the Olympics, Gould et al. (1998) concluded that the confi-dence of successful athletes needed to be deeply embedded on a rational, emotional, and subconscious level.

Because confidence is crucially important, yet seemed to be lacking in the Women's National Ice Hockey team at previous world championships, it became an important focus in preparation for the Olympics. However, having awareness of the importance of confidence is one thing; knowing how to foster its growth on a rational, emotional, and subconscious level is something else altogether. There is no simple blueprint to follow, but the sport psychology literature offers guidelines on how to go about it, and as is the case in any applied setting, those guidelines need to be adjusted with some creativity to the specific situation. Being trained in a science practitioner model requires that interventions be based as much as possible on tested theoretical models. Trying to derive interventions from theory allows for the formulation of educated guesses in the absence of definite suggestions from the research, which limits the likelihood of a "shot in the dark." To borrow an old expression, "nothing is more practical than a good theory."

A number of theoretical models guided the interventions used with the women's Olympic team. Bandura's theory of self-efficacy and collective efficacy (1986, 1997) guided the development of interventions for developing individual and team confidence. Csikszentmihalyi's theory of flow (1990), which has considerable support from the applied sport psychology literature (S. A. Jackson, 1992, 1995, 1996), strongly influenced interventions developed for achieving optimal experience with the athletes. In a nutshell, the goal of any intervention is to help the athlete achieve optimal performance. Athletes refer to this as being "in the zone;" Csikszentmihalyi describes it as being in flow. Being in flow is a special experiential state, characterized by a balance of challenge and skills, clear goals, unambiguous feedback, a merging of action and awareness, concentration on the task at hand, experience of a sense of control, the absence of self-evaluation, and often a transformation of time. Performing in such a flow state is not only deeply rewarding, but also increases the chances of achieving the desired outcome.

However, achieving a state of flow at the Olympic games is a difficult process for a number of reasons. Nations place extreme importance on this international competition, and these high expectations transfer to the athlete. One mistake, one loss can take a team out of contention for the coveted medals. Because of this, athletes are exposed to incredible levels of stress, which makes it especially difficult to balance challenge with skill and merge action with awareness. Stress is generally characterized as the perceived imbalance between the demands of a situation (the challenge) and the response capabilities (the skills one brings to the table). So in order to achieve flow and handle stress effectively, it is important to maintain that challenge/skill balance, which means increasing skills and/or lowering the perception of the challenge. The nature of Olympic competition requires athletes to perform in what Giges (1998) calls the "here and now" (or merging thought and action) in order to perform at their highest level. Sometimes psychological barriers prevent the athlete from being in the here and now, and so the intervention is geared towards removing those barriers. This is how two players on the Olympic team describe such an experiential state of optimal performance:

> It's exciting, I remember being so charged and excited and ready to get back out on the ice, and very, you know, like I said, very focused, I guess very focused on myself, but in a good way, like focused on, you know, being in tune with my thoughts, being in tune with everything that I am doing, every move I am making, every pass I am making, choices I make, being very in tune and very energized I guess, and it is one of those things where if you make a bad play it just doesn't matter, you know, or if you make a good play you are building on it, and you are excited about it, and it takes you through the next shift, but you know, not letting any negative things bother you, [not] being frustrated about not scoring a goal. It wasn't a negative thing that day, you know, whereas another day, if you hit the post twice,"you dumb idiot, what are you thinking," but for me it was like "wow look at what I can do, now let's do some more."

> When I play the best . . . , when I am in that zone . . . I am the most confident and it's like "go ahead, shoot on me." You are just like "you are not going to score," you know. You just feel like you are having control over everything.

It is the authors' contention that the ideal performance at the Olympics occurs when such an experiential state is achieved. As these statements indicate, being in the zone, being in flow, is equivalent to having high confidence, which explains the focus on confidence in psychological preparation for the Olympics.

The Confidence of the Olympic Team

The following quotes from three team members illustrate how players on the Women's Olympic Ice Hockey Team perceived the team's confidence level going into the games:

> I think we had all the confidence in the world that we could beat them.

> You know, I would say our confidence was good, but for the

gold medal game, it wasn't even in question, like, we just knew that we were going to [win], like, it is hard to describe that people didn't seem that nervous. It was just like "we are just going to go and do it," and that was it. So, I mean that is a whole different level of confidence that goes beyond, you know, kind of like that scale.

I think it was very high. I think that everyone, especially with the way that January had gone, were, you know, I think that, even though we didn't win all the games in January, I think by the third period, we just felt that we were the stronger team, we were the better team, and we had gotten to the point where we knew that we were better—and so I think we, you know, were entirely confident that we were going to be successful in our goal and that, I think, is the key thing, is the difference between that team going into that tournament and us going into like every other tournament that we have played in. It is just knowing, knowing that we were going to win, not that we could win, but that we were going to, going to win.

These quotes amply describe the team's level of confidence, a confidence that seems deeply embedded on a rational, emotional, and subconscious level. This is similar to the level of confidence shown on the men's volleyball team in 1984 (Beal, 1985). Furthermore, this deeply seated confidence also distinguished this Women's Olympic Ice Hockey team from previous World Championship teams:

I think the biggest thing, the most important thing was just the attitude and confidence of going in and knowing that, like "we're gonna win, we're gonna win this," and we never had that—at least I have never felt that before with the team. And we've never had this, you know, the same amount of cohesiveness, either, this kind of always, ah, been some fragments that didn't work, some pieces of the puzzle that didn't really fit, whether it be certain players, or several times it's been coaches . . . that kind of hindered the whole team progress, so there was always just some areas that were never quite right. I mean, most recently at the Worlds, I remember, before going into the overtime . . . , feeling scared, being afraid to lose, and afraid to feel that feeling of losing and with this team it was like the opposite. I mean, the whole week, I'd be just visualizing like being on the, you know, receiv-

ing the gold medal. I mean, I wouldn't even be thinking about it
—that's when I'd be visualizing, and visualizing like winning and
winning, and what it would feel like to win, and not, God, I can't
even really remember ever thinking, like "What if we lose?" or it
pops in your head, that vision of, like, that feeling, like it never,
I never felt it, that whole time we were there, which is amazing.
It is quite, it is a big contrast. And a lot of that is just this team
knew how to win . . .

How Did This Sense of Confidence Develop?

The previous quote highlights not only the level of confidence the team felt,
but also the difference from the level of confidence during the world championships. Furthermore it starts addressing some of the reasons for being so
confident.

For Bandura (1986) the sources of confidence are performance accomplishments, modeling, verbal persuasion, and emotional arousal. The importance of performance accomplishments cannot be underestimated. Early on
in the Olympic year, the coaching staff decided to play the Canadian team as
much as possible, knowing that with the team's talent level, it was only a matter of time before games would be won. This strategy clearly paid off:

> . . . having played Canada 15 times was a huge factor, because
> they went from having this kind of aura about them, of being,
> you know, the best team, and championship team, and, too, you
> know, after you play them several times, you're "hey, they are just
> another team, and we are [just] as good," and it kind of took
> them off that pedestal, which they had put themselves on . . .
> . . . with each win that we had against Canada, and even each loss,
> because it was a one-goal loss, you know, or it was a really close
> game, ah-m, so each victory or each close loss kind of built that
> confidence up . . .

So not only winning, but winning the close games the team played during
the pre-Olympic tour fueled confidence. The two teams played each other 13
times during the pre-Olympic tour, with Canada winning seven and the United
States winning six (the goal differential was exactly the same). This more general sense of confidence was built on being confident in all areas of the game:

> . . . we were very confident in our power-play, very confident in
> penalty killing, [the] goal tenders we had absolutely the most con-

fidence in them, and I think they felt the confidence from the net out, you know, like they had confidence in their defenders, and the forwards, our forechecking. I thought nobody forechecked better than our team, we were quick to jump on the puck . . . . every aspect of the game I felt like we were confident in.

Having success continued at the Olympics, as the United States defeated Canada in the final game of the round-robin format 7-4 after being down 1-4 with 12 minutes to go. This stunning performance accomplishment seemed to cement the players' beliefs in themselves:

. . . in the first Canadian game, I think that just put us like "wow —we can do anything,"'cause we were down and if you looked at everything, we were down by so many goals and with the amount of time we had left, I mean, that was almost like we had never done it before, scored so many goals against Canada in that amount of time and we were just like "awesome," like the team pulled together.

. . . Coach Smith called the time out at the right time, and he was just like "you guys," you know, he gave us a little pep talk, and we just pulled together, and all of a sudden, the goals were just amazing. And I think that was just like "wow," you know, "if we can do this we are winning the medal," like that was it, I mean we weren't going to let them take it away from us after that.

Besides success in games, another source of confidence, particularly for female athletes, seems to be the perception of mental and physical readiness (Jones, Swain, & Cale, 1991). There is a fine line between doing too much and not doing enough, and often there is a tendency to do too much, to cram right before the game. Again, this is where experienced coaching is crucial. For the Atlanta Olympians, coaching actions such as providing excellent physical/technical training, facilitating mental preparation and training, organizing the environment, and preparing and protecting athletes from distractions enhanced their performance (Gould et al., 1998). All these factors can be summarized under preparation, and the hockey players consider this comprehensive preparation crucial as well:

Preparation, all the physical preparation, mental preparation, just everything, I think that that was the big thing . . .

I felt like we were so prepared that once we got there, we just had to stick to our game plan, and we could do it . . .

I think we were totally prepared. And you know I think that is why we were able to stay so loose, just 'cause we knew we were ready and that was it.

I don't think we could have been any more ready. . . . I think like the mental part of the game, we were ready, we couldn't have been any more mentally prepared than we were, and physically we couldn't have gotten any stronger. I mean, it was all—it came down to just us going out there and wanting it more. I mean, we did everything we could to prepare ourselves.

Performance accomplishments are usually considered the most important source of confidence. As these quotes indicate, preparation and the perception of being prepared played an important part in the development of confidence for these athletes. Whereas physical preparation was achieved by adhering to a strict strength and conditioning program on and off the ice, mental preparation basically followed Bandura's (1986) recommendations for developing confidence by using modeling and verbal persuasion and managing the perceptions of emotional arousal. Hardy (1997) points out that these three aspects often get neglected in the pursuit of optimizing confidence. He considers this a mistake, a mistake the Olympic team tried to avoid.

Modeling to Build Confidence

Modeling has been used in various forms. Although the sport psychology literature generally recommends using a model that is roughly equal in skill and equal in gender as the most effective model (Hardy et al., 1996), a useful model for the Olympic team proved to be the boxing legend Muhammad Ali. In one of the pre-Olympic sport psychology meetings, the team watched the Oscar-winning documentary "When We Were Kings," which, in a very dramatic way, tells the story of the fight for the World Heavyweight Championship in boxing between George Foreman and Muhammad Ali in 1974. Ali, who won an Olympic gold medal in 1960, was the underdog going into this fight. Not only was he the underdog, but the common perception from media and boxing experts also was that he would be badly beaten in the ring, because George Foreman was so young, so strong, and at the pinnacle of his career. In previous bouts Foreman had destroyed Joe Frazier and Ken Norton, two fighters who had beaten Ali. One quickly realizes that nobody believed in Ali. So here is the first similarity as a useful model for the women's team: the fact that one is considered an underdog, and that all bets are on the other team. The next useful aspect of this movie is why Ali wants to win this fight. Very eloquently, he addresses the importance of having a higher purpose, that it is not just winning itself that helps him be motivated, but that winning will enable him to do something positive for his people. Successful coaches consider having a higher purpose crucial for team cohesion and success (P. Jackson & Delahanty, 1995). After watching this sequence in the movie, the players were asked why it was personally important for them to win the gold medal in Nagano, to write this down, and then to share it with their teammates. This became a powerful emotional moment for the players, because the reasoning they shared was very personal. Sharing this contributed to the understanding that all the players were pursuing the same goal and deepened their already existing commitment to this goal.

> I have never, ever in my life been on a team where more than, where we, where every single person on that team was more committed and every single person from the first person to the 20th person was focused on that one thing and wanted it that much, never in my life, like I have never seen more, more than 20 people, like sacrifice themselves and give up their own selfishness for the team, and I felt we had total, complete perfection in that, I really do.

In addition, Ali provides in the movie an excellent example of the power of positive self-talk. For months, by constantly praising himself and his own ability, he literally convinces himself and his staff that he can beat Foreman. Obviously this overt verbal cockiness was not the model we wanted to emulate, because this seemed rather unique to Muhammad Ali and would not have fit well with the rather modest style of our players. The teaching point, and the modeling, nevertheless hold up, because the key issue here is the importance of managing one's self-talk, particularly the covert self-talk. We believe this is particularly important with elite female athletes. Our applied experience shows that female athletes can be their own worst enemy, because their self-talk can be extremely self-critical. Ali was an important role model here, as his self-talk was always motivational and/or instructional, but never judgmental. The players learned to manage their self-talk effectively in crucial situations:

> . . . it was in the gold medal game . . . . and I was just going out on the power-play, and there wasn't even really much time left, I think maybe only 30 seconds or something, and I'd been not feeling confident at all back there, and so I said to myself, like "This is crazy." I am like "I can do this, I know how to do this," and we scored.

Verbal persuasion as a source of confidence can be used effectively by the coach as well as by teammates, as the following player quotes indicate:

> . . . he did like an amazing job of that, and . . . . it was contagious, you know, just a contagious feeling throughout the team, and he made us like believe in ourselves, whether it was player X taking a face-off and how important, she'd had to do it late in the game, or you know whether it was player Y on the point, like he instilled like that confidence in each player and then we were on, it was, I thought he did a really, really good job of that, individual, and then as a team, we just, like I said, we gained that confidence.

> . . . just players, throughout the year, like making little comments, you know, like, positive little comments that they may not even know were positive or that makes you feel good . . . . and it could have the greatest effect on you.

The other important aspect from a modeling perspective is that Ali did not just use his self-talk effectively, but he also prepared and planned extremely well for the fight. Modeling was also used in the form of imagery in preparation for the Olympics, this time with the athletes as their own model. Regular group imagery sessions were conducted throughout the preparation phase. Imagery scripts that addressed all aspects of the Olympic experience (from traveling to processing to playing the different games themselves) were prepared and utilized. Not only did these imagery exercises help with building confidence, but they also facilitated cohesion, as the players enjoyed the quiet time together and the exercises provided a common language to handle some of the stress of the Olympics. Video highlights of the team, intermixed with clips from the movie, provided another modeling perspective, and such clips were repeatedly used at crucial points during the Olympic tour to nurture confidence and to reemphasize key concepts of mental toughness.

Ali is also a great role model for managing emotional arousal effectively. The movie provides some insight into his emotional state leading up to the fight and during the fight itself. After the first round of the title bout, Ali realizes that his plan has not worked out, and he now has to deal with the fear of losing, the fear of getting destroyed in the ring. He does this by accepting fear and then drawing on his own resources to conquer it. The lesson here is that even the best and mentally toughest athletes can experience anxiety in competition (in Ali's case, it is actually fear, because the threat to his physical well being was quite real). As Hardy (1997) stated, cognitive anxiety does not necessarily have to be detrimental to performance. We wanted to make sure that our athletes understood that at some time during the Olympics they would be afraid and that this feeling was quite all right. Being afraid is part of the deal. Cognitive anxiety itself is not the problem; the problem is being afraid about being afraid, and when that happens, it is difficult to utilize coping resources. The goal here was to prepare our players for experiencing, accepting, and channeling effectively the whole range of emotions during the Olympics. Again, the coach played a crucial role in this, not only from the perspective of modeling confidence and emotional management himself, but also from the point of monitoring and influencing the players' emotional state:

> . . . emotionally I think Coach really kept us, like pretty loose . . . , we knew that it was intense, I mean how could we not know that it was an intense experience, you know? Coach kind of has the unique gift of keeping things light, but at the same time not lose focus or seriousness. And so I think from an emotional standpoint we knew that something big was going to happen, and I felt like we were relaxed enough to just go with it, and mentally, mentally I think going over there I was pretty apprehensive, but once we got to the village and started practicing and stuff, I think that everybody kind of just knew what we had to do, you know, so I think mentally we were really prepared too. I think we were totally prepared. And you know I think that is why we were able to stay so loose.

During the brief literature review of this chapter, the connection between cohesion and confidence was raised. Obviously, cohesion was a big part of the Olympic preparation, and a discussion of the effort to facilitate the formation of a cohesive team would be the topic of another chapter. Suffice it to say that all efforts at building cohesion culminated in the concept of the "inner circle." The inner circle consists only of the players and the staff; everybody else (media, agents, friends, family, etc.) was part of the outer circle. During the Olympics, only the inner circle can help the athletes achieve their performance goals; everything else is viewed as a distraction that interferes with performance. This concept of the inner circle grew out of the team-building sessions with the players and was symbolized by the players' wearing a simple bracelet, cut from a piece of rope and tied to each other's wrist. This inner-circle bracelet became a powerful metaphor for the inner state of the team, symbolizing strength, trust, unity, and total commitment to a common goal. The reason this concept is mentioned here is that from the players' perspective, cohesion had a profound influence on confidence:

> [Cohesion]—I think it was everything, I think it was the performance. . . . I think it just made us solid, it made us have that confidence in, in your teammates, which gives you the confidence that you can win, you know. I mean, you don't question what's going on, you don't question the coaches, you don't question who's on the ice. It is just a complete confidence that you are a group of 20 and anybody can do the job, and, it'll run perfectly.
>
> I think it affected us in a positive manner, just because I felt confident in everybody, and I believed in everybody, and I trusted everybody, and I feel that's the way our team worked.

The other aspect of cohesion that warrants mentioning in connection with confidence is the importance of role clarification, acceptance, and performance. Not only does role acceptance foster cohesion, but it also influenced confidence (Feltz & Bandura, 1989). Again, the role of the coach here is crucial, and a masterful job was accomplished by the head coach in giving each player an important role and communicating the importance of that role to the team:

> Coach made you feel that your role on the team was just as important as anybody else's. He made you feel that whatever your role on the team was, it was a key—a key role.

From a sport psychology perspective, this process of role appreciation was facilitated by making sure that highlight videos included all these roles. Also, the players shared their appreciation of each other's role in written form, by letting each individual teammate know what she contributed to the team, thus culminating in each player's receiving positive feedback from 19 teammates.

Summary

This chapter briefly discussed the importance of confidence in an Olympic gold-medal-winning team and the efforts made to foster this level of confidence. In reflecting on the importance of confidence, it is important to keep in mind that successful performance at the Olympics is "a complex, multifaceted, fragile, and long-term process that requires extensive planning and painstaking implementation" (Gould et al., 1998, p. 11).

Confidence and mental preparation are only two aspects of this multifaceted process. Mental preparation and confidence alone do not lead to optimal performance and gold medals, but they are crucial ingredients in this complex process.

References

Bandura, A. (1986). *Social foundations of thought and action: A social cognitive theory.* Princeton, NJ: Van Nostrand.

Bandura, A. (1997). *Self-efficacy: The exercise of control.* New York: Freeman.

Beal, D. (1985). *Spike: The story of the victorious U.S. volleyball team.* San Diego, CA: Avant Books.

Csikszentmihalyi, M. (1990). *Flow: The psychology of optimal experience.* New York: Harper & Row.

Feltz, D. L., & Bandura, A. (1989). *Individual and team confidence in hockey: Final report.* USOC Sports Science NGB Grants Program.

Giges, B. (1998, September). *Psychological barriers to excellence in sport performance.* Paper presented at AAASP conference, Hyannis, MA.

Gould, D., Eklund, R. C., & Jackson, S. A. (1992a). 1988 U.S. Olympic wrestling excellence I: Mental preparation, precompetitive cognition and affect. *The Sport Psychologist, 6,* 358-382.

Gould, D., Eklund, R. C., & Jackson, S. A. (1992b). 1988 U.S. Olympic wrestling excellence II: Thoughts and affect occurring during competition. *The Sport Psychologist, 6,* 383-402.

Gould, D., Guinan, D., Greenleaf, C., Medbery, R., Strickland, M., Lauer, L., Yongchul, C., & Peterson, K. (1998). *Positive and negative factors influencing U.S. Olympic athletes and coaches: Atlanta Games assessment: Final report.* USOC Sport Science and Technology Grant Project.

Gould, D., Weiss, M. R., & Weinberg, R. S. (1981). Psychological characteristics of successful and non-successful Big Ten wrestlers. *Journal of Sport Psychology, 3,* 69-81.

Haberl, P. (2000). *Peak performance at the Olympics: An in-depth psycho-social case study of the 1998 US Women's Ice Hockey Olympic Team.* Unpublished doctoral dissertation, Boston University.

Hardy, L. (1997). Three myths about applied consultancy work. *Journal of Applied Sport Psychology, 9,* 277-294.

Hardy, L., Jones, G., & Gould, D. (1996). *Understanding psychological preparation for sport: Theory and practice of elite performers.* Chichester, England: John Wiley & Sons.

Jackson, P., & Delahanty, H. (1995). *Sacred hoops: Spiritual lessons of a hardwood warrior.* New York: Hyperion.

Jackson, S. A. (1992). Athletes in flow: A qualitative investigation of flow states in elite figure skaters. *Journal of Applied Sport Psychology, 4,* 161-180.

Jackson, S. A. (1995). Factors influencing the occurrence of flow state in elite athletes. *Journal of Applied Sport Psychology, 7,* 138-166.

Jackson, S. A. (1996). Toward a conceptual understanding of the flow experience in elite athletes. *Research Quarterly for Exercise and Sport, 67,* 76-90.

Jones, G., Swain, A. B. J., & Cale, A. (1991). Gender differences in precompetition temporal patterning and antecedents of anxiety and self-confidence. *Journal of Sport and Exercise Psychology, 13,* 1-15.

Mahoney, M. J., & Avener, M. (1977). Psychology of the elite athlete: An exploratory study. *Cognitive Therapy and Research, 1,* 135-141.

McFarlane, B. (1994). *Proud past, bright future: One hundred years of Canadian women's hockey.* Toronto, Canada: Stoddart.

Weinberg, R. S., & Gould, D. (1999). *Foundations of sport and exercise psychology* (2nd ed.). Champaign, IL: Human Kinetics.

Williams, J. M., & Krane, V. (1998). Psychological characteristics of peak performance. In J. M. Williams (Ed.), *Applied sport psychology: Personal growth to peak performance* (3rd ed., pp. 158-170). Mountainview, CA: Mayfield.

CHAPTER 12

Working With Individual Team Sports: The Psychology of Track and Field

Ralph A. Vernacchia

Abstract

This chapter addresses the salient aspects of "working with an individual team sport" such as track and field. An overview of the culture, politics, and mentality of track and field are provided in order to give prospective sport psychology consultants a better understanding of the social and performance climate of track and field. Emphasis is also placed on team dynamics, with particular focus on the importance of social support and recognition of gender differences as key components of the team-building process. Additionally, a track and field-specific model for the design and implementation of educational mental-skills training program is presented.

Although the phrase "individual team sports" appears to be an oxymoron, it is, in fact, a statement of reality for many sport psychology consultants who work with sports such as swimming, tennis, track and field, and golf. It must be kept in mind that coaches of these sports consider their sport to be a team sport, that is, one in which the cumulative individual performances of their athletes determine the team success. On the other hand, it is generally difficult for the athletes of individual team sports to comprehend the collective effect their performances may have on their teammates as well as on "team" success. The sport of track and field is an excellent example of an individual team sport whose performance outcomes can be affected by psychosocial influences and activities such as team building, group cohesion, and social support, as well as mental skills training.

This chapter takes a sport-specific approach to examining the world of the individual team sport, because many of the psychosocial dynamics present in the sport of track and field are similar to other individual team sports.

Furthermore this chapter will provide practical guidelines for sport psychology consultants to follow when developing and implementing mental-skills training programs for track and field coaches and athletes.

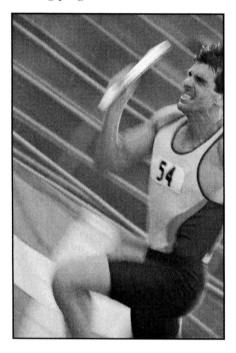

Though coaches of individual team sports work with athletes who perform individually, they still consider the athletes and their performances an integral part of a team.

Understanding the World of Track and Field

Track and field is a very diverse sport in terms of task demands because there can be as many as 23 events contested in a track meet, depending on the level of competition. Many athletes compete in several events throughout the course of a track meet, and it is not uncommon for athletes to compete in 3 or 4 events per competition. As a result of the diversity and availability of competitive opportunities for athletes, track and field is a sport of participation and self-improvement.

Participation

One of the most disruptive factors in the team-building process is the issue of playing time. In many sports, opportunities to participate are limited; for example, a basketball team may be composed of 12 to 15 team members, but only 5 start the game and perhaps as few as 7 actually play throughout the course of the game. Other team members may be designated as "practice" players. Most athletes join a team to play and test their skills in competitive athletic situations, not just to practice, so playing time can be a critical impediment to team building.

As a result of the diversity of track and field events (i.e., sprinting, hurdling, running, race walking, throwing, jumping, vaulting), there is an event for every athlete and an athlete for every event. In most cases there are not enough athletes on a track and field team available to participate in all 20 or more events, especially because it is desirable for each team to have at least 3 athletes in each event. The greater the number of athletes a team has per event strongly influences their ability to score points and win team competitions. In track and field, as in other sports, this dimension of a team-performance profile is known as team depth.

The very real prospect of inclusion in the competitive setting is a very attractive aspect of track and field; it provides a purpose and reward for the hard work and training that is necessary to prepare oneself for competition. Most important, it gives the athlete a legitimate opportunity to test him- or herself in competitive settings free of the politics that sometimes surround team selection and playing time. Performance in track and field can be measured in very objective ways (i.e., time and distance), and through direct competition there is very little room for controversy when it comes to the selection process. Track and field athletes, for the most part, have the opportunity to earn their place on a team through their individual performance efforts.

In many cases the coach-athlete relationship in the sport of track and field is enhanced as a result of the many competitive opportunities available to athletes. Track and field coaches can serve in more of an advisory role with their athletes, because the coach does not determine who gets to play or participate —in track and field it is the athlete, by virtue of training and performance outcomes, who determines whether he or she will be selected for competitive opportunities if such a selection needs to be made. Therefore, communication between coach and athlete is heightened, and athletes tend to tell their coaches what they "really" think and feel rather than what they think the coach wants to hear. It is easier for the coach to be an advocate for his or her athletes once the barriers of selective participation in competitive opportunities have been removed.

Self-Improvement

Track and field athletes soon come to realize that they have total control over the outcomes of their performances. It is this sense of control combined with the objective measurement of performance that provides an atmosphere of performance security as well as performance goals that are very motivating to pursue. Even if an athlete does not win a particular competition, he or she can improve on a personal best and experience a personal victory.

Personal victories motivated by self-improvement are at the heart of the athlete's motivational fuel for success in track and field. The Olympic motto "Swifter, Higher, Stronger" best typifies the attitude of self-improvement that results from athletes' comparing themselves to themselves as they strive to be the best in each and every competition. Track athletes soon learn to run "their race" rather than to compare themselves to others—they know they have no control over their opponent's performance and that they have total control over their own performance.

Track and field is essentially a developmental sport, and self-improvement is at the heart of an athlete's personal, psychological, and physical development. Conscientious practice and training in their specific event provides athletes with the opportunity to develop themselves on a daily basis, thereby preparing themselves for future competitive performances. For the track and field coach and athlete, the relationship between quality training and enhanced performance is crystal clear.

Team Dynamics

One of the paramount concerns of most coaches is the willingness and ability of their athletes to attain team and individual goals. It seems reasonable that individual athletes cooperating with teammates would most easily accomplish these goals, and for this reason team "chemistry" is a major concern of coaches, and track and field coaches are no exception. In terms of team performance, coaches strive to blend the talents and strengths of individual team members into a force that is greater than the sum of their individual performances—this is referred to as team synergy (Yukelson, 1997).

The coach is the chief architect of a cohesive team. Coaches define cohesiveness as a bonding of diverse individuals toward common goals (Brennan, 1995). McGuire (1998), himself a track and field coach, states that synergistic performance will "occur as a result of skilled leadership, displaying great knowledge and understanding driven by empathic caring, and applied with experienced wisdom" (p. 139). Ultimately, the coach's ability to build a cohesive team is dependent on several factors, including understanding the team-building process; engineering the team climate, culture, and environment; leading through influence; communicating with athletes and other members of the coaching staff; and providing leadership for the staff (McGuire, 1998). These factors as well as the issue of gender differences related to team building and communication will be addressed in the next several sections of this chapter.

Team Cohesion

Recognizing that all groups are not teams, coaches attempt to create team synergy by employing a variety of team-building strategies and techniques directed toward establishing team cohesion (Hardy & Crace, 1997). Team cohesion is "a dynamic process that is reflected in the tendency for a group to stick together and remain united in pursuit of its goals and objectives" (Carron, 1982, p. 124). In addition to contributing to team cohesion, team-building strategies and techniques can address the following related components of effective teams: team structure (role clarity and acceptance, leadership, and conformity to standards), team environment (togetherness and distinctiveness), and team processes (sacrifices, goals and objectives, and cooperation; Prapavessis, Carron, & Spink, 1996).

In terms of team building, it is important for coaches to target the type of cohesion they would like to develop within their team—task cohesion, social cohesion, or both. Task cohesion involves members of a group working together to achieve a specific and identifiable task, such as team goals and performance objectives (Carron, 1982; Cox, 1998; Gill, 2000). Social cohesion concerns itself with friendship issues (i.e., whether team members like each other and enjoy each other's company), as well as other interpersonal concerns such as social-emotional support (Cox, 1998; Gill, 2000).

In general, the research literature regarding cohesiveness and athletic performance (Gill, 2000) provides the following guidelines for coaches:

1. Cohesiveness increases motivation and commitment to team goals, and hence cohesiveness should enhance performance; however, if emphasizing team goals detracts from the recognition and encouragement of individual contributions and goals, performance may suffer.

2. High social cohesion or interpersonal attraction could detract from performance if team members sacrifice performance goals and task-interaction strategies to maintain friendship patterns. However, social support and encouragement from teammates have potential positive effects on performance if individuals are committed to performance and task goals.

3. Cohesiveness, defined and measured as attraction-to-group, is positively related to success in interactive team sports.

4. Cohesiveness may influence performance, but the evidence indicates that success enhances cohesiveness, and there are only weak indications that cohesiveness affects performance.

These findings regarding the relationship of cohesiveness to team performance would tend to suggest that (a) coaches should establish strong social intrateam cohesion to facilitate communication and cooperation among team members, and (b) the primary emphasis of the team should be on task cohesion, that is, adherence to team and individual performance goals and behaviors (Vernacchia, McGuire, & Cook, 1996).

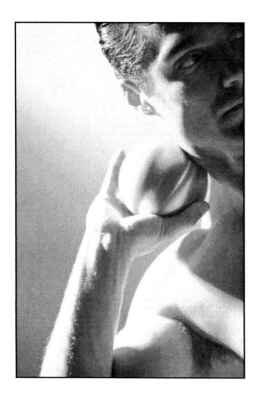

As part of an individual team sport, each athlete must concentrate on his or her own physical conditioning and motor-skill development.

Cohesion and Team Building in Track and Field

Task cohesion and mastery. Track and field, by the very nature of the training and practice patterns of team members, requires a tremendous commitment to task cohesion, that is, toward the mastery of physical conditioning and motor-skill development that will ultimately result in effective individual performance within the team context. Mastering the execution and performance of movement skills in challenging competitive situations is the key to athletic performance in any sport.

Effective track and field performances result from taking one's ability and improving it through conscientious practice until it is equal to meeting the demands of the performance setting. Once an athlete can master an event and meet the demands of competition, sport becomes more enjoyable as the athlete becomes proud of his or her preparation and ability to reach team and personal performance goals. Individual pride as a result of hard work and task or event mastery can form a sense of collective competency among team members as they view their ability to undertake performance challenges.

Social cohesion and social support. It is important to remember that track and field practice sessions are individualized by events, and that although team members can practice at the same time as their teammates, they practice in different places. Distance runners may be on a run miles away from the track, and sprinters and hurdlers may be training on the track, while other athletes are strength training in a weight room, and field-event athletes may be training at an area located away from the track. Because track and field has such a strong inclination toward individualized practice orientation, many athletes train by themselves at various times during the day. The only time the team truly comes together is during competition, and even then, events are scheduled at different times throughout the duration of a track meet.

Because the social interaction opportunities for team members are limited during practice, team-building activities that develop social cohesion are important in track and field because they provide opportunities for team members to interact. These activities can include team meals, team social gatherings and activities, and team travel, as well as training activities such as group runs, group warm-ups, and team stretching and flexibility.

Most important, team activities designed to build social cohesion set the stage for generating the social support necessary to succeed in demanding track and field training and performance settings. Practicing in isolation; training in various climatic conditions; enduring injuries, poor performances or performance slumps; and balancing life and academic demands are but a few of the elements that can ultimately influence and/or interfere with the attainment of team and personal performance goals. Social support can facilitate the team-building process by providing team members with opportunities for social and emotional growth within the demanding context of the athletic arena (Rosenfeld & Richman, 1997).

Social support strategies and interventions can be helpful in the team-building process by promoting communication among team members and between team members and the coach, which in turn provides team members with a sense of physical and mental well-being and satisfaction with team experiences and leadership (Rosenfeld & Richman, 1997). As an intervention strategy, social support can provide the encouragement and resources necessary to reduce stress, combat overtraining and burnout, increase feelings of well-being, and overcome feelings of isolation associated with training (Rosenfeld & Richman, 1997).

Support, encouragement, care, and concern provided by teammates and coaches are essential in providing both the motivational fuel necessary to overcome adversity and the meaning for an athlete's quest for performance excellence. If team members can provide each other with social support, "they are likely to enhance their communication and share a deeper commitment to the team goals and team vision of success" (Rosenfeld & Richman, 1997, pp. 140-141).

Rosenfeld and Richman (1997) suggest the following strategies for the various types of social support that can be used in the team-building process:

Listening Support (team members feel someone can listen to their concerns and problems without giving advice and being judgmental): nonjudgmental active listening between team members and team staff regarding the stress of training and performance demands; providing group social events for coaches, staff, and athletes so they can "step out of sport" and their roles within the team and relate to each other on a more personal level; promoting informal contacts among team members, the coaching staff, and other support personnel; structuring the practice environment to convey warmth, friendliness, and acceptance.

Emotional Support (providing team members with a feeling of care and concern, that someone is on their side): stressing the importance of emotional support to team leaders so they may provide and model such support for team members; encouraging emotional support for injured athletes; encouraging the staff to be available to team members away from practice; making the services of a sport psychologist available to the team and staff.

Emotional Challenge Support (team members feel that others challenge them to evaluate their attitudes, values, and feelings; a type of support is provided by friends, parents, and coaches, not teammates): using team meetings, team talks, and team themes, etc., to help team members focus, or in some cases refocus, their emotional energy on their performance; having teammates provide verbal encouragement in challenging training and performance situations.

Task Appreciation Support (acknowledging the efforts of team members and displaying an appreciation for their work ethic): coaches and teammates reinforcing and affirming the training effort of teammates who are striving to master their event skills through conscientious and dedicated practice; providing awards ceremonies to reward improvement as well as outstanding performances; using the media to convey the value and significance of performance accomplishments.

Task Challenge Support (team members are made to feel that others will challenge them to challenge themselves in terms of improving their ability and performance effectiveness): Coaches' and teammates' providing positive reinforcement and information/corrective feedback to challenge athletes to enhance training and performance efforts; using technology (i.e., videotaping, etc.) to provide feedback and enhance performance; encouraging athletes to accept task challenge as a team responsibility and norm.

Tangible Assistance Support (provision of support resources): Providing training equipment and facilities, economic support when appropriate (scholarships), and support for travel to competitions.

Personal Assistance Support (assistance with lifestyle needs unrelated to sport): Teammates' helping each other with academic interests (peer advising), transportation to social events, errands, personal needs during injury rehabilitation, etc.

The Team-Building Process

Leadership, team standards, and expectations. The coach's philosophy regarding the program that they oversee is an essential but often overlooked key component of the team-building process. Foundational beliefs are essential to an efficient athletic program and team. As the team leader, the coach must clearly define and express to the staff and team members the team's mission, rules, and guiding principles for the conduct of all those persons who are a part of the team (Vernacchia et al., 1996).

The foundational beliefs of an athletic program or team represent the educational values, ideals, and standards upon which resulting attitudes and behaviors are predicated, evaluated, rewarded, and sanctioned. This is especially important when conflict arises within a team, because personal agendas and self-centered concerns can often lead to misinterpretation regarding the original mission and purpose of team goals (Vernacchia et al., 1996).

Most sport leaders are well focused on the purpose of their programs (performance outcomes) but often lack a well-defined coaching philosophy that reflects their vision for the governance, conduct, and success of their teams. A clearly communicated, ethically sound, and educationally mature philosophy of sport and coaching is a prime prerequisite for success in the team-building process goals (Vernacchia et al., 1996).

One of the most overlooked teams in the team-building process is the "staff" team. It is essential that all members of the coaching staff be "on the same page" with regard to team standards, mission, goals, and strategies. A leadership adage states that "water runs downhill." Team cohesion is preceded by staff cohesion, that is, a unified effort among all staff members that is directed toward maximizing team and individual performance.

Many unsuccessful teams are characterized by the "teams-within-teams" orientation (i.e., defense vs. offense, events vs. events, etc.), which promotes intrateam competition rather than intrateam cooperation and support. Teams can self-destruct from within if they cannot cooperate and focus their resources on interteam competition. As McGuire (1998) stated:

> It is the responsibility of the head coach to provide effective leadership and influence to insure that the staff team is a highly "performing" team, supportive of one another and delivering a consistent message to the rest of the athletes and team. Anything less than this will sow the seeds of destruction, predictably undermining the overall team building effort. (p. 148)

Team-building stages. In general, groups of individuals experience four distinct stages in the team-building process: forming, storming, norming, and performing (Tuckman, 1965; Tuckman & Jensen, 1977).

The forming stage is the stage of team selection, the establishment of team and individual goals, and the assignment of roles and responsibilities to each team member. The storming stage is a stage of role acceptance and conflict usually resulting from team members' unwillingness to conform to the team's mission, philosophy, and their assigned roles and responsibilities. Once team members accept their individual roles on a team and understand how each person's role contributes to the team's overall effectiveness, the team enters the norming stage. It is in this stage that the team begins to work together by performing their assigned roles. The final team-building stage, the performing stage, is one of silent communication among and between team members, who interact harmoniously to realize team goals and performance outcomes. This is the stage of the team-building process in which team members respect and trust each other and their collective ability to accomplish performance tasks and challenges goals (Vernacchia et al., 1996).

Team-building problems can arise in each of these stages if the guidelines for team selection, conflict resolution between the coach and team members or among team members, and specifically, the criteria for participation or "playing time" in team competitions are not clearly explained and adhered to. Essentially, the athlete wants to be a part of a team that he or she can trust and a team process that treats him or her fairly.

Team climate. Coaches are very concerned about creating a team climate or atmosphere that will foster, encourage, and insure successful performances. Although there can be no guarantees regarding performance outcomes, it is generally accepted that a "team culture" that emphasizes team spirit and unity can lead to successful athletic performances (Watson, 1989).

Coaches can create a team climate that fosters a successful team culture by building commitment, rewarding competency, and maintaining consistency (Martens, 1987). Commitment can be built by involving players in defining team goals, recognizing that team goals are compatible with individual goals, giving players responsibilities that they can accommodate, demonstrating superior skill and knowledge of the sport, and treating each player with respect (Martens, 1987; Watson, 1989).

Competency can be rewarded by taking time to notice it; rewarding it promptly; rewarding excellent performance and effort, not outcomes that are beyond the athlete's control; and teaching players to reward each other (Martens, 1987; Watson, 1989). Consistency can be maintained by developing a sound coaching philosophy, taking a long-term rather than a short-term perspective, and sticking with a well-thought-out plan when adversity occurs (Martens, 1987; Watson, 1989).

Communication. The ability of the coach to effectively communicate and demonstrate his or her ideas and philosophy regarding the team's mission and goals is an essential prerequisite for the team-building process and, ultimately, for the team's success. To this end, Anshel (1997) stated, "No matter how brilliant a coach might be in planning strategy and knowing the technical aspects of his or her game, success depends on the coach's ability to communicate effectively with the athletes" (p. 209).

As stated previously, athletes seek the security of fairness, care, and concern in the team environment, and the coach is the gatekeeper of the team process. The coach must be able to communicate, through word and action, his or her care, concern, and support for each athlete's committed training and performance efforts. This is essential in the sport of track and field because the coach-athlete relationship tends to have more of an advisory nature, which emphasizes social interaction, technical knowledge, and task mastery. McGuire (1998) suggested the following basic communication guidelines for enhancing the team-building process:

1. Always communicate with those below you as you would wish to be communicated with by those from above you! This is no more than the "Golden Rule" applied to issues of communication within a team.
2. Seek to have important communications within a team provided in a REGULAR, CONSISTENT, and THOROUGH manner.
3. Always take care of the "Bottom Rung." (p. 148)

Coach-athlete communication can always take place in a respectful way, a way that emphasizes the positive and provides feedback to improve on the negative. Coaches need to remind athletes that any feedback that they might provide is about the athlete's performance or behavior and not about the athlete personally.

Anshel (1997) suggested that coaches use the "sandwich approach" in providing constructive feedback in sport. Essentially this approach begins by providing the athlete with a positive statement regarding his or her training or performance efforts and then providing the corrective, informative, or prescriptive feedback necessary to successfully perform a specific skill or behavior in the future. In the final stage of this approach, the coach compliments the athlete on the improvement he or she has made and encourages the athlete to sustain his or her efforts until the performance skill or behavior is mastered.

Because communication is a two-way process (speaking and listening) between individuals, it requires a high degree of concentration to be successful (Yambor, 1992). The key to effective communication is to be a good listener, that is, one who is empathic and nonjudgmental, one who listens with an "open mind" (Yambor, 1992). The listener must also be aware of nonverbal communication such as body language (posture, gestures, eye and facial movements, physical appearance), spatial relationships (distance between one another, arrangement of the environment, etc.), and paralanguage (vocal components of speech, such as pitch or tempo; Yambor, 1992). The listener must determine not only what is being said but also what is "really" being communicated. How we say what we say is just as important or sometimes more important than what we say.

On the other hand, it is important for the speaker to communicate in a clear, consistent, and complete manner (Yambor, 1992). The speaker's communication should be direct rather than hinting or implying something; it should not contain hidden agendas, but should separate fact from opinion, focus on one thing at a time, use "I" statements that take ownership rather than "we" statements that deflect ownership, and use verbal and nonverbal statements that match (Yambor, 1992). Most important, the speaker should obtain feedback from the listener to determine if the communication was clearly understood (Yambor, 1992).

Because conflict is a "natural" part of the team-building process (the storming stage), it is also important for coaches and athletes to be trained in conflict-resolution methods. Intrateam conflicts usually stem from miscommunication and misinterpretation of team standards, norms, roles, and goals; how the coaching staff and team members respond to intrateam conflict can make or break a team. Coaches and athletes should recognize that intrateam conflicts (coach-athlete, athlete-athlete) are a natural part of the team-building process, hence the following adage, "A ship is safe in the harbor, but that's not what it's built for." Vernacchia and his colleagues (1996) suggested the following steps for resolving conflict in team settings:

1. Speak to the team member(s) in a neutral setting away from the coach's office (i.e., go for a walk, have lunch together, etc.);
2. Address conflicts directly, honestly, and expeditiously;
3. Listen to all sides of the issue/problem and then present your concerns;
4. Repeat the issue/problem until the emotional component has been diffused;
5. Relate the issue to team standards and goals so that the athletes can determine the effect of particular behaviors and attitudes upon team

performance and cohesion;

6. Negotiate a solution to the conflict/problem that is acceptable to all parties, thus facilitating a win-win outcome;

7. Have an objective party (i.e., athletic director, coach, sport psychologist, etc.) facilitate conflict resolution if necessary;

8. Explain to the athletes that conflict is healthy when dealt with in a mature, respectful, and open manner and that it can enhance understanding and communication among team members and the coach;

9. Use informal (conversation) or formal (meetings) follow-up sessions to evaluate the effectiveness of the established solution(s). Meet again to discuss the problem/issue if necessary. (pp. 52-53)

Diffusing or stabilizing the emotional component of communication is extremely important in conflict-resolution situations. Checking one's mood before verbally interacting with others can go a long way in building and maintaining open, honest, and effective communication with others.

Gender differences. Because it is an accepted practice that track and field coaches coach both men and women within the context of their training programs, it is relevant here to address gender differentiated preferences toward leadership, training, learning, and performance. For example, in summarizing the relationship of coaching behavior to athlete preference and satisfaction, Carron and Hausenblas (1998) proposed the following: Male athletes had a high preference for more training and for autocratic and social support from their coaches; female athletes had a high preference for democratic behavior from their coaches; as the coach's training and positive feedback increased, athlete satisfaction increased; and coach-female athlete relationships were poor when the coach was perceived as providing less positive feedback and more autocratic behavior than preferred.

Sport psychology researchers have identified gender-different responses to sport participation in a variety of psychosocial domains, including emotional response (anxiety), motivation (causal attributions, participation, and achievement motivation), aggression, leadership preference, confidence, and communication (Anshel & Hoosima, 1989; Bjorkqvist, Osterman, & Kaukianinen, 1992; Chelladurai, Haggerty, & Baxter 1989; Eccles & Harold, 1991; Feltz, 1988; Flood & Hellstedt, 1990; Gill, 1988; Gill & Dzewaltowski, 1988; Gould, Feltz, & Weiss, 1985; Jones & Cale, 1989; Jones, Swain, & Cale, 1991; Lirgg, 1991; Martens, Burton, Vealey, Bump, & Smith, 1990; Rainey & Cunningham, 1988; Shaw & Gouran, 1990; White, 1993; Wood, 1993). It should be noted that although the sport psychology research literature highlights certain gender differences among male and female athletes, male and female athletes tend to become less differentiated as they approach and attain elite status in their sport. The majority of gender differences are to be found among athletes at the entry and developmental levels and stages of athletic participation, when athletes, particularly female athletes, are learning to overcome gender socialization and stereotypical attitudes and expectations.

Tuffey (1996a, b) interviewed 14 collegiate cross-country and track coaches regarding gender differences and coaching styles. Although this is a limited survey in terms of the number of coaches surveyed, the study can provide valuable qualitative feedback regarding the gender differences and preferences related to coaching track and field athletes. As a result of her research, Tuffey (1995) proposed the following practical implications for coaching male and female athletes:

Treat each athlete as an individual. Respond to the individual needs and wants of each athlete, as there is more variability between athletes than between males and females.

Similarities outnumber the differences. While males and females differ in many respects and may need to be approached differently in some situations, it needs to be recognized that they are more similar than different.

Expect and accept different emotional reactions. Male and female athletes are different emotionally and may react differently to the same situation. Coaches need to be aware of and accepting of these differences.

Look beyond outward expression. Coaches must be careful when "reading athletes" based on outward behavior alone, as they may not show the emotions they are really feeling. Both males and females (but especially males) have a tendency to suppress certain emotions.

Extra effort may be needed to break down barriers put up by male athletes. Males tend not to openly communicate verbally or non-verbally—coaches need to work at getting through their tough exterior.

Be aware that females tend to value a relationship with the coach. They want and expect more from the coach than the Xs and Os of coaching. A unique relationship with the coach is an important aspect of her athletic experience. It is possible that males may also need more from the coach but just don't express it.

Be careful not to abuse or misuse power with female athletes. The tendency of females to be very coachable and to want to please the coach gives power to the coach and exposes her to potential abuse.

Emphasize performance goals to a greater extent with males. Because males have a tendency to focus on winning, coaches may need to stress personal perform-ance goals to facilitate the opportunity of experiencing personal success.

Attempt to take pressure off regarding expectations. This seems especially impor-tant for females as they tend to feel the expectations of their coach, parents, and others.

Be aware that females may overwork in practice. Because of the female tenden-cy to want to please, she may push too hard in a practice session to please the coach. She may also overwork to maintain her position on the team.

Athletes can be used as a vehicle for social change. Coaches can model or facili-tate behavior that goes against "gender socialization."

Coach education can increase awareness of gender-related differences and dispel myths. Scientific knowledge of gender, while it may not always impact coach behav-ior, seems to be important to enhance coaches' understanding of their male and female athletes. This knowledge can aid in the development of accurate expectations that, in turn, can facilitate coach behavior and coach-athlete inter-action. A caution is that awareness and understanding should be flexible, not judgmental. And, above all else, coaches need to respond to the individual. (pp. 23-24)

Mental Skills Training for Track and Field Athletes

Once the proper social and training environment has been established for an athlete who is a member of an "individual team" sport such as track and field, the next step is to focus on the identification of specific mental skills that will enhance track and field performance. Although this is the next step in the process of effective athletic performance, it is not the first step: The first step lies in the willingness of the athlete to mentally and physically prepare for competition.

Mental skills training can enhance both the training and performance process and goes hand in hand with the athlete's physical preparation. At all times during the practice phase of the athletes' development, it is crucial that they realize that the purpose of their training is to perform. As in all sports, it is easy for an athlete to lose performance focus while training and fall in love with the ritual and routine of practice. Not only does this orientation lead ath-letes to overtrain, but it also creates the athlete who trains and trains and then gets in the track meet and trains some more.

Mental skills training can help athletes develop a love affair with performing, because it helps the athlete master the emotional component that is missing from training settings. The ability to adapt to the psychologically distracting and disrupting aspects of athletic competition is an essential prerequisite for effective athletic performance. In terms of competitive effectiveness, elite athletes distinguish themselves from nonelite athletes by moderating worry and performance anxiety, utilizing their concentration abilities, remaining self-confident, focusing on internal kinesthetic imagery, and maintaining motivation and personal meaning (Mahoney, Gabriel, & Perkins, 1987).

In an effort to ascertain the importance of mental training to the performance of elite athletes, Orlick and Partington (1988) surveyed 235 members of the 1984 winter and summer Canadian Olympic teams. They found several elements related to successful performance in all sports, including quality training (the athletes' ability to train with the highest degree of quality utilizing mental imagery and personal commitment in order to give their best effort in reaching performance goals); clear daily goals (the athletes set clear daily goals for practice as well as performance settings); imagery training (used to enhance training, perfect motor skills, make technical correction, and image successful competitive performances); simulation training (training in practice as if they were performing in the competitive situation—replicating in practice the specific protocols that are used in the performance setting, including equipment, time schedules, and routines); mental preparation for competition (including a precompetition plan, a competition focus plan, a competition evaluation plan, and a distraction-control plan; Orlick & Partington, 1998). Orlick and Partington stressed the fact that all of these mental preparation skills and behaviors have to be learned, mastered, and refined into personal plans for success in competition.

Researchers (Gould et al., 1998) have also surveyed members of the 1996 United States Olympic team to determine factors that influence performance in world-class competitive settings. Gould et al. (1998) found the following factors to be critical considerations in preparing athletes for international competition such as the Olympic Games: distraction control; adherence to physical and mental preparation plans; optimal physical training that avoids overtraining; mental preparation to cope with the stress of world-level competition; team cohesion and harmony; a sound coach-athlete relationship, including team coaches as well as personal coaches who are experienced in guiding athletes in high-performance settings; support personnel including administrators, massage therapists, physicians, athletic trainers, personal coaches, and sport psychology specialists; team training/residency programs or training camps for the athletes so they can make the transition into high-performance settings; and planning to deal with family and friends, media, and sponsors.

When athletes were asked what they would do differently if they could perform again at the Games, they indicated that they would: focus more on sport psychology and mental preparation; get more rest and not overtrain; optimize their physical training and preparation; plan and be better prepared to deal with distractions; focus more on team cohesion; and focus more on relaxation and stress management (Gould et al., 1998). Gould and his associates concluded that

> successful Olympic performance is a complex, multifaceted, fragile, and long-term process that requires extensive planning and painstaking implementation. It seldom happens by chance and can easily be disrupted by numerous distractions. Attention to detail counts, but must also be accompanied by flexibility to deal with numerous unexpected events. (p. 11)

Mental Training and Track and Field

Mental preparation has become an integral part of the track and field athlete's training program. Today, sport psychologists advise track and field athletes at all levels and even travel with national teams to international competitions as members of the team's support staff (McGuire & Balague, 1993; Nideffer, 1989). Psychological skills programs for track and field athletes have been designed, implemented, and evaluated for athletes at various levels of their development in order to enhance performance and increase participation satisfaction (Belciug, 1992; Blumenshtein & Knudadov, 1983; Ebbeck & Weiss, 1988; Fairall & Rodgers, 1997; Jermolajova, 1988; Krane & Williams, 1994; Neubauer, Miller, & Vernacchia, 1994; Poole & Henschen, 1984; Vernacchia, 1998; Vernacchia, Austin, VandenHazel, & Roe, 1992). In 1992, an entire issue of the Track and Field Quarterly was devoted to addressing the theme "Maximizing athletic performance and personal growth through applied sport psychology" (Vernacchia & Gordin, 1992).

As early as 1973, prominent American track and field coaches such as Dr. LeRoy Walker, the 1976 USA head Olympic track coach, addressed the importance of developing a "psychological winning edge" (Walker, 1977). More recently, sport scientist and two-time Olympic javelin champion Ruth Fuchs (1990) pointed to the importance of psychological skill development as it relates to high achievement in track and field, when she stated:

> The closer the physical level of achievement of the athletic competitors, the more the degree to which the level of psychological achievement components has been developed becomes the decisive factor for winning. The cognitive-emotional-motivational activity aspects that are necessary for high athletic achievement become continuously available with great certainty if they are stable and firmly established psychological personality traits. (p. 16)

Members of the 1992 United States Olympic track and field team reported using a variety of mental preparation techniques, including goal setting, concentration, imagery/visualization, relaxation training, refocusing/coping, thought control, prayer, and breathing control (McGuire & Balague, 1993). Vernacchia, McGuire, Reardon, and Templin (2000) interviewed 15 former U.S. Olympians (1984-1996) and found the following mental skills and attitudes to be associated with athletic success: fun and enjoyment (participation vs. mastery), perseverance/persistence, mental imagery/visualization, patience, confidence, dream goals, cognitive restructuring, and the ability to overcome obstacles (injuries, socialization, legal issues).

In an extensive psychological study of elite track and field athletes, Ungerleider and Golding (1990, 1992) surveyed 633 Olympic hopefuls who qualified to participate in the 1988 U. S. Olympic track and field trials. In addition to the survey, interviews were conducted with 16 randomly selected athletes. Survey and interview findings (Ungerleider & Golding, 1990) indicated that: 1) 85% of the athletes practiced some form of mental practice; 2) field athletes were more likely to use mental practice strategies than were track competitors; 3) more educated athletes, those who dream about competition, and those who daydream about competition were also more likely to report mental practice before their event; 4) working with a sport psychologist was related to engaging in mental practice; 5) among field athletes, Olympians were more likely than non Olympians to visualize during competition; 6) the Profile of Mood States (POMS) inventory results indicated that athletes who reported making highly stressful sacrifices to train for the U.S. Trials also reported relatively high levels of anxiety, depression, anger, fatigue, and confusion, and low levels of vigor. These athletes also displayed relatively high levels of overall mood disturbance; 7) athletes who reported higher stress in the year before the U.S. Trials were also more likely to be injured during that year; 8) Olympians were less depressed, and showed less overall mood disturbance than non-Olympians; 9) athletes who have a coach report more athletic stress than those who don't train with a coach; 10) 92% of the study's elite athletes have experienced injury at some time in their life, and nearly half reported being injured one to three months prior to the 1988 U.S. Olympic Trials; 11) the average amount of time all injured athletes took for recovery was 36 days; 12) athletes who had been injured at some time in their lives were more anxious than those who had never been injured; 13) injured athletes were no less likely to be selected for the Olympic team than were non-injured athletes; 14) track athletes tended to assess their physical and mental efforts to cope with injury relatively favorably, marathoners relatively unfavorably; 15) athletes training with a coach assessed their physical coping strategies toward injury in the year before the Trials more favorably than did those without a coach, and those athletes were also less likely to report frustration; 16) athletes who used imagery to heal injuries sustained during the year before the Trials were more likely to qualify for the Olympic team than injured athletes who did not use imagery; 17) athletes with higher athletic and life event stress levels before the Trials were also more likely to use imagery to cope with injury with favorable results for their performance; 18) athletes who trained long and hard (training hours per month) perceived their sacrifice as relatively stressful; this group also reported a greater commitment to making the team; 19) athletes who described their coach as more emotionally supportive—that is, the coach was described as reliable, caring and trustworthy—reported greater commitment to making the team than those with less supportive coaches; 20) number of training hours seems to be associated with a particular style of coping (longer training hours with logical analysis, information seeking, and problem solving); 21) older and more educated athletes were more likely to report logical analysis and problem solving in coping with the stress of training for the Trials.

In a specific analysis of the psychological characteristics of elite junior (ages 16-19) male and female throwers in a field event, Reardon (1991) reported that although both genders were similar in their profiles, differences that did exist favored the psychological stability (state and trait anxiety, achievement motivation, mood states, and self-concept) of the female throwers. Reardon (1991) observed "that 'elite' athletes may be elite performers but that they are in fact very ordinary in terms of their susceptibility to psychological pressures" (p. 3629).

Periodization of Mental Skills Training

In recent years sport psychology practitioners have become more interested in organizing mental skills training in a way that would complement the physical training patterns of athletes who are preparing themselves for peak performance. This is critical in track and field because it is important that an athlete's training culminate in the ability to perform at his or her highest level during the final stages of the competitive season when the most important championship meets occur (conference, NCAA, Olympic Trials, World Championships, Olympic Games, etc.).

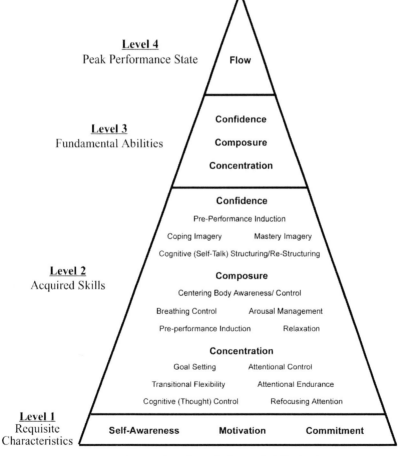

Level 4
Peak Performance State — **Flow**

Level 3
Fundamental Abilities
- Confidence
- Composure
- Concentration

Level 2
Acquired Skills

Confidence
Pre-Performance Induction
Coping Imagery   Mastery Imagery
Cognitive (Self-Talk) Structuring/Re-Structuring

Composure
Centering Body Awareness/ Control
Breathing Control   Arousal Management
Pre-performance Induction   Relaxation

Concentration
Goal Setting   Attentional Control
Transitional Flexibility   Attentional Endurance
Cognitive (Thought) Control   Refocusing Attention

Level 1
Requisite Characteristics
Self-Awareness   Motivation   Commitment

*Figure 1. Hierarchy of psychological skill development
leading to achievement of flow state*

Autumn	Winter	Spring	Summer
Transition Phase of Training (Oct. -Nov.)	General Phase of Training (Nov. - Dec.)	General - Specific Phase of Training (Jan. - Feb. - Mar.)	Competition Phase of Training (April. - Sept.)
Composure Skills Breathing Centering Arousal management Relaxation Formal/informal biofeedback - Heart rate - Respiration - GSR **Concentration Skills** Goal setting Attention drills	**Composure Skills** Continue practice Integrate into lifting and throwing practices **Concentration Skills** Attention controls Attentional endurance Refocusing attention Begin cognitive (self-talk) training	**Composure/Concent ration Skills** Practice becomes more specific; competitive setting Simulate meets/competition **Confidence Skills** Cognitive programming specific to meets Develop pre-perform-ance routine Practice mastery imagery Practice coping imagery utilizing composure, concentration, and confidence skills Skills are becoming more integrated into day-to-day mental/ physical routines	Concentration/com-posure/confidence abilities are honed and refined by competitive experiences Pre-performance routine becomes more "automatic" and is integrated into the athlete's cogni-tive/physical/behav-ioral schema Emphasis is on holistic approach aimed at flow state during championship competitions

Table 1. Psychological Periodization (Reardon & Gordon, 1992)

In line with the work of Moore and Stevenson (1991, 1994, 1995), Figure 1 illustrates a periodization model for psychological skill development that can lead to a peak performance "flow state" (Gordin & Reardon, 1995; Reardon, 1992a, b; Reardon & Gordin, 1992). The focal point of this model is the progressive development and mastery of the mental attributes of concentration (the act or process of directing one's attention to a single object; see chapter 9, which focuses on concentration in sport), composure (a calmness of mind, body, bearing, and appearance), and confidence (a state of mind or conscious-ness marked by certainty of one's abilities and ease and freedom from doubt;

see chapter 11, which elaborates upon confidence in team sports; Reardon, 1992a, b; Reardon & Gordin, 1992). The development and mastery of fundamental and advanced mental skills is necessary for effective or "flow-state" performance in important competitions—"physical and psychological training cycles are focused toward a simultaneous peak, thereby providing the optimal opportunity for peak performance" (Reardon & Gordin, p. 22).

Reardon and Gordin (1992) have outlined a timetable for psychological periodization that would correspond and dovetail with an annual physical training cycle for track and field athletes (see Table 1). Gordin and Reardon's (1995) model of psychological periodization views mental skills training from an educational rather than an interventionist perspective. Mental skill mastery can empower track and field athletes to perform at their highest level: "Ideally, by 'big-meet' day there is nothing left to do but relax and 'let it happen.' All the preparation is done and flow has been programmed into the person's conscious and unconscious minds" (Reardon & Gordin, p. 22).

Summary

Working with individual team sports requires the sport psychology consultant to creatively "individualize" educational performance-enhancement programs and interventions. Successful consultants recognize that the key to the effective implementation of educational and interventionist programs is eliciting and securing the support of the coach who designs, supervises, and implements the athlete's training program. As stated at the beginning of this chapter, coaches in a variety of "individual" team sports take an individualized team approach to their sport. They recognize individual differences in the development and performance of athletic talent and allow for the flexibility within training programs to accommodate these differences; in essence, they recognize that individuals learn and perform differently.

In addition to recognizing individual differences among athletes, it is extremely important to recognize that talent development and effective athletic performances do not occur in a social vacuum. Athletes are humans, not machines, and they need social contact in a supportive environment that is geared toward self-improvement and mastery of athletic skills and personal self-growth via athletic participation.

Creating an environment that will lead to team synergy can provide team members with a task focus in a socially supportive training and performance environment that cultivates success. This is especially true in track and field because athletes often practice alone, with training partners, or in small groups. To this end, coaches must be sensitive to the team-building stages, and particularly with the communication aspect of the coach-athlete relationship. Sport psychology consultants can help coaches construct a supportive team environment by addressing the importance of the various aspects of building cohesive teams, including task cohesion and mastery, social cohesion and social support, leadership (team and staff), team climate, conflict resolution, and gender differences.

Finally, a periodized mental skills program can serve to enhance the performance effectiveness of track and field athletes not only because it complements and enhances physical training but also because it helps athletes adapt, cope, and plan for success in highly charged and often distracting competitive environments. Enjoyment, fun, and success in athletic performance settings are often the results of the mastery and application of mental and physical skills developed through conscientious training and applied with committed effort.

References

Anshel, M. H. (1997). *Sport psychology: From theory to practice* (3rd ed.). Scottsdale, AZ: Gorsuch Scarisbrick Publishers.

Anshel, M., & Hoosima, D. (1989). The effect of positive and negative feedback on causal attributions and motor performance as a function of gender and athletic participation. *Journal of Sport Behavior, 12,* 119-130.

Belciug, M. P. (1992). Affective consequences of personally-perceived success and failure in high-performance competitive athletics. *South African Journal for Research in Sport, Physical Education, and Recreation, 15,* 1-10.

Bjorkqvist, K., Osterman, K., & Kaukiainen, A. (1992). The development of direct and indirect aggressive strategies in males and females. In K. Bjorkqvist (Ed.), *Of mice and women: Aspects of female aggression* (pp. 51-64). New York: Macmillan.

Blumenshtein, B. D., & Khudadov, N. A. (1983). Psychological essentials of technical improvement in speed-strength events in track and field. *Teoriya i Praktika Fizicheskoi Kultury, 4,* 47-49.

Brennan, S. J. (1995). *Competitive excellence: The psychology and strategy of successful team building* (2nd ed.). Omaha, NE: Peak Performance.

Carron, A. V. (1982). Cohesiveness in sport groups: Interpretations and considerations. *Journal of Sport Psychology, 4,* 123-138.

Carron, A. V., & Hausenblas, H. A. (1998). *Group dynamics in sport* (2nd ed.). Morgantown, WV: Fitness Information Technology.

Chelladurai, P., Haggerty, T., & Baxter, P. (1989). Decision style choices of university basketball coaches and players. *Journal of Sport and Exercise Psychology, 11,* 201-215.

Cox, R. H. (1998). *Sport psychology: Concepts and applications* (4th ed.). Boston: WCB/McGraw Hill.

Ebbeck, V., & Weiss, M. (1988). The arousal-performance relationship: Task characteristics and performance measures in track and field athletics. *The Sport Psychologist, 2,* 13-27.

Eccles, J., & Harold, R. (1991). Gender differences in sport involvement: Applying the Eccles' expectancy-value model. *Journal of Applied Sport Psychology, 3,* 7-35.

Fairall, D. G., & Rodgers, W. M. (1997). The effects of goal-setting method on goal attributes in athletes: A field experiment. *Journal of Sport and Exercise Psychology, 19,* 1-16.

Feltz, D. (1988). Gender differences in the causal elements of self-efficacy on a high avoidance motor task. *Journal of Sport and Exercise Psychology, 10,* 151-165.

Flood, S., & Hellstedt, J. (1990). Gender differences in motivation for intercollegiate athletic participation. *Journal of Sport Behavior, 14,* 159-167.

Fuchs, R. (1990). Striving for success: Personality development and high achievement in athletics. *New Studies in Athletics, 5,* 16-20.

Gill, D. L. (1988). Gender differences in competitive orientation and sport participation. *International Journal of Sport Psychology, 19,* 145-159.

Gill, D. L. (2000). *Psychological dynamics of sport and exercise* (2nd ed.). Champaign, IL: Human Kinetics.

Gill, D. L., & Dzewaltowski, D. (1988). Competitive orientations among intercollegiate athletes: Is winning the only thing? *The Sport Psychologist, 2,* 212-221.

Gordin, R. D., & Reardon, J. P. (1995). Achieving the zone: The study of flow in sport. In K. P. Henschen & W. F. Straub (Eds.), *Sport psychology: An analysis of athlete behavior* (3rd ed., pp. 223-230). Longmeadow, MA: Mouvement.

Gould, D., Feltz, D., & Weiss, M. (1985). Motives for participation in competitive youth swimming. *International Journal of Sport Psychology, 6,* 126-140.

Gould, D., Guinan, D., Greenleaf, C., Medbery, R., Strickland, M., Lauer, L., Chung, Y., & Peterson, K. (1998, June). *Positive and negative factors influencing U.S. Olympic athletes and coaches: Atlanta Games assessment.* Colorado Springs, CO: United States Olympic Committee.

Hardy, C. J., & Crace, R. K. (1997). Foundations of team building: Introduction to the team building primer. *Journal of Applied Sport Psychology, 9,* 1-10.

Jermolajora, N. (1988). Psychological problems of jumpers. *Modern Athlete and Coach, 26,* 11-13.

Jones, G., & Cale, A. (1989). Precompetition temporal patterning of anxiety and self-confidence in males and females. *Journal of Sport Behavior, 12,* 183-195.

Jones, G., Swain, A., & Cale, A. (1991). Gender differences in precompetition temporal patterning and antecedents of anxiety and self-confidence. *Journal of Sport and Exercise Psychology, 1,* 350-358.

Krane, V., & Williams, J. (1994). Cognitive anxiety, somatic anxiety, and confidence in track and field athletics: The impact of gender competitive level and task characteristics. *International Journal of Sport Psychology, 25,* 203-217.

Lirgg, C. (1991). Gender differences in self-confidence in physical activity: A meta-analysis of recent studies. *Journal of Sport and Exercise Psychology, 8,* 294-310.

Mahoney, M. J., Gabriel, T. J., & Perkins, T. S. (1987). Psychological skills and exceptional athletic performance. *The Sport Psychologist, 1,* 181-199.

Martens, R. (1987). *Coaches' guide to sport psychology.* Champaign, IL: Human Kinetics.

Martens, R., Burton, D., Vealey, R., Bump, L., & Smith, D. (1990). The development of the Competitive State Anxiety Inventory-2 (CSAI-2). In R. Martens, R. Vealey, & D. Burton (Eds.), *Competitive anxiety in sport* (pp. 117-190). Champaign, IL: Human Kinetics.

McGuire, R. (1998). Team issues and considerations. In M. Thompson, R. A. Vernacchia, & W. Moore (Eds.), *Case studies in applied sport psychology: An educational approach* (pp.139-156). Dubuque, IA: Kendall/Hunt.

McGuire, R., & Balague, G. (1993). Profiling the '92 Olympic track & field team. *American Athletics, 5,* 26-27.

Moore, W. E., & Stevenson, J. R. (1991). Understanding trust in the performance of complex automatic sport skills. *The Sport Psychologist, 5,* 281-289.

Moore, W. E., & Stevenson, J. R. (1994) Training for trust in sport skills. *The Sport Psychologist, 8,* 1-12.

Moore, W. E., & Stevenson, J. R. (1995). Trust in the performance of sport skills. In K. P. Henschen & W. F. Straub (Eds.), *Sport psychology: An analysis of athlete behavior* (3rd ed., pp. 393-403). Longmeadow, MA: Mouvement.

Neubauer, J. P., Miller, L., & Vernacchia, R. A. (1994). A prospective view on mental practice research: The logic and use of the cognitive rehearsal technique of creative concentration. *Applied Research in Coaching and Athletics Annual,* 119-141.

Nideffer, R. M. (1989). Psychological services for the U.S. track and field team. *The Sport Psychologist, 3,* 350-357.

Orlick, T., & Partington, J. (1988). Mental links to excellence. *The Sport Psychologist, 2,* 105-130.

Poole, R. C., & Henschen, K. (1984). Brigham Young's psychological program for women's cross country and track. *Scholastic Coach, 53,* 52-53, 73-75.

Prapavessis, H., Carron, A. A., & Spink, K. S. (1996). Team building in sport. *International Journal of Sport Psychology, 27,* 269-285.

Rainey, D., & Cunningham, H. (1988). Competitive trait anxiety in male and female college athletes. *Research Quarterly for Exercise and Sport, 59,* 244-247.

Reardon, J. (1991). Psychological characteristics of elite junior male and female throwers. *Track Technique, 114,* 3627-3629.

Reardon, J. (1992a). Learning how to "go with the flow." *American Athletics, 4*, 54-55.

Reardon, J. (1992b). The three c's of success: Concentration, composure, confidence are the key. *American Athletics, 4*, 48-50.

Reardon, J., & Gordin, R. (1992). Psychological skill development leading to a peak performance "flow state." *Track and Field Quarterly, 92*, 22-25.

Rosenfeld, L. B., & Richman, J. M. (1997). Developing effective social support: Team building and the social support process. *Journal of Applied Sport Psychology, 9*, 133-153.

Shaw, T., & Gouran, S. (1990). Group dynamics and communication. In J. Dahnke & S. Clatterbuck (Eds.), *Human communication: Theory and research.* Belmont, CA: Wadsworth Publishing.

Tuckman, B. W. (1965). Development sequence in small groups. *Psychological Bulletin, 63*, 384-399.

Tuckman, B. W., & Jensen, M. A. C. (1977). Stages of small group development revisited. *Group and Organizational Studies, 2*, 419-427.

Tuffey, S. L. (1995). *Coaching athletes: Does (Should) gender make a difference?* Unpublished manuscript.

Tuffey, S. L. (1996a). Coach perceptions of psychological characteristics and behaviors of male and female athletes and their impact on coach behaviors (women athletes, men athletes, coaches, gender differences). *Dissertation Abstracts International, 56*(8), 3051A. (University Microfims No. AAT96-44130).

Tuffey, S. L. (1996b). *Psychological characteristics of male and female athletes and their impact on coaching behavior.* Unpublished manuscript.

Ungerleider, S., & Golding, J. M. (1990). *Elite athlete project research questionnaire: A report to the Athletics Congress on elite track and field athletes.* Eugene, OR: Integrated Research Services.

Ungerleider, S., & Golding, J. M. (1992). *Beyond strength: Psychological profiles of Olympic athletes.* Dubuque, IA: Wm. C. Brown.

Vernacchia, R. A. (1998). Competitive refocusing and the performance of USA international junior elite track and field athletes. *New Studies in Athletics, 13*, 25-30.

Vernacchia, R. A., Austin, S., VandenHazel, M., & Roe, R. (1992). The influence of self-hypnosis on the performance of intercollegiate track and field athletes. *Applied Research in Coaching and Athletics Annual*, 77-91.

Vernacchia, R. A., & Gordin, R. (Eds.). (1992). Maximizing athletic performance and personal growth through applied sport psychology. *Track and Field Quarterly, 22,* 1-78.

Vernacchia, R. A., McGuire, R., & Cook, D. (1996). *Coaching mental excellence: "It does matter whether you win or lose...".* Portola Valley, CA: Warde.

Vernacchia, R. A., McGuire, R., Reardon, J., & Templin, D. Psychosocial characteristics of Olympic track and field athletes. *International Journal of Sport Psychology, 31,* 5-23.

Walker, L. (1977). Producing that psychological winning edge. *Track and Field Quarterly, 77,* 15-17.

Watson, L. K. (1989). Building team culture. *Coaching Volleyball, 3,* 27.

White, S. (1993). The relationship between psychological skills, experience, and practice commitment among collegiate male and female skiers. *The Sport Psychologist, 7,* 49-57.

Wood, J. (1993). The relationship between psychological skills, experience, and practice commitment among collegiate male and female skiers. *The Sport Psychologist, 7,* 49-57.

Yambor, J. (1992). Improving communication skills and building cohesiveness. *Track and Field Quarterly, 92,* 32-34.

Yukelson, D. (1997). Principles of effective team building interventions in sport: A direct services approach at Penn State University. *Journal of Applied Sport Psychology, 9,* 73-96.

ABOUT THE EDITORS

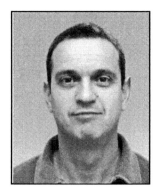

Ronnie Lidor is a senior lecturer at both the Zinman College of Physical Education and Sport Sciences at the Wingate Institute and at the Faculty of Education at Haifa University (Israel). Dr. Lidor has published about 70 articles, book chapters, and proceedings chapters in English and Hebrew. He is the senior editor of the books Sport Psychology: Linking Theory and Practice, (1999), and The World Sport Psychology SourceBook (3rd ed.), (2001), published by Fitness Information Technology (FIT). From 1997 to 2001 Dr. Lidor served as President of the Israeli Society for Sport Psychology and Sociology (ISSPS), and since 1997 he has been a member of the Managing Council of the International Society of Sport Psychology (ISSP). In 2001 he was elected as the Secretary General of the ISSP, and he has been the editor of Movemen-Journal of Physical Education and Sport Sciences (Hebrew) since 1999.

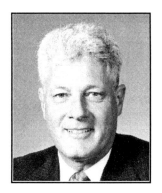

Keith Page Henschen is a professor in the department of exercise and sport science at the University of Utah, with an area of expertise in the psychosocial aspects of sport. Dr. Henschen received a PED degree from Indiana University in 1971 and has been a member of the University of Utah faculty for the past 30 years. His research interests include the psychology of performance, use of psychological interventions in sport, and sport psychology for special populations. Dr. Henschen has co-authored four textbooks and published approximately 200 articles, 24 chapters of books, and 5 monographs. He has directed 40 doctoral dissertations and 20 masters' theses. He is a frequent research presenter and conference speaker with over 400 presentations. He has served as president (1997-98) of the American Alliance of Health, Physical Education, Recreation, and Dance (AAHPERD), and he is currently president of the International Society of Sport Psychology (ISSP). Dr. Henschen has consulted with numerous world-class, professional, and elite level athletes as well as six National Governing Boards (NGB's) for the United States Olympic Committee. He has worked with teams in track and field, biathlons, gymnastics, skiing, and speed skating. Dr. Henschen also works with numerous college and professional teams in a variety of sports.

ABOUT THE CONTRIBUTORS

Gloria Balague started her professional career in her native Barcelona (Spain), working with elite athletes and teams at the National Sports Research Center and teaching at the College of Physical Education. She obtained her doctorate in clinical and social psychology at the University of Illinois in Chicago, where she is currently a clinical assistant professor. Her main research interests are achievement motivation and elite level performance for athletes and coaches. She has worked with numerous elite level athletes, including USA Track & Field, USA Gymnastics, and USA Field Hockey. She has been actively involved with international sport psychology, serving as vice-president of the International Society of Sport Psychology (ISSP) from 1989-1993 and acting as the current president of the Division of Sport Psychology in the International Association of Applied Psychology (IAAP).

Cal Botterill has been a sport psychology consultant to a number of world championship teams and athletes. He has worked with four National Hockey League teams, including the 1994 Stanley Cup champion New York Rangers, and has attended six Olympic Games. Cal completed his PhD at the University of Alberta and has been a professor at the University of Winnipeg for the past twenty-two years. He is a "teaching excellence" award winner and has made over 200 international, national, and regional presentations in sport, psychology, medicine, education, and business. Cal has published more than 100 articles, chapters, videotapes, audiotapes, and books. He has served as mentor to numerous graduate students and has recently been active in distance learning, international tele-courses, and online education.

David L. Cook is president of San Antonio-based Mental Advantage, Inc., a performance enhancement firm that bridges the gap between the sports and business arenas. He also serves as Director of the Mindset Academy at both the Water Chase Golf Academy in Ft. Worth and the Academy of Golf at La Cantera in San Antonio (site of the Texas Open). Dr. Cook is a speaker for the prestigious Zig Ziglar Corporation and serves as the mental training coach for the San Antonio Spurs in the NBA. He has counseled over 100 professional golfers, as well as elite performers from the NBA, NFL, Major League

Baseball, Olympics, and collegiate national championship ranks. His business clients have included Compaq, Heinz, American Express, Bristol-Myers Squibb, Texas Instruments, Bayer Corp., the Associates, State Farm Insurance, and many others. He is the former director of applied sport and performance psychology at the University of Kansas where his peers elected him president of the Sport Psychology Academy in 1992. During his twelve-year tenure at the University of Kansas, he counseled over 1500 athletes and coaches.

Dr. Paul Dennis is the development coach for the Toronto Maple Leafs of the National Hockey League. He assists the athletes with psychological skills training and consults with the coaching staff on issues pertaining to group dynamics and team-building. Dr. Dennis began his association with the Toronto Maple Leafs in the mid-1980s as head coach of the Maple Leaf-owned Toronto Marlboros (part of the Ontario Hockey League) and became the Leafs' video coach in 1989. He was the video coach/applied psychologist for the club before receiving his current role. Dr. Dennis has a PhD in sport psychology from the University of Western Ontario, where he studied under Dr. A. V. Carron. He is also an adjunct professor in the kinesiology department at York University.

Dr. Paul Estabrooks is an assistant professor in the department of kinesiology at Kansas State University. He received his PhD in 1999 at the University of Western Ontario where he studied under the supervision of Dr. A. V. Carron. Dr. Estabrooks currently teaches courses in group dynamics and leadership. His research has focused on the relationships between group environments, physical activity, and sport performance. Most recently, he has applied team-building techniques to community coalitions for the promotion of physical activity. His research has been published in a number of scientific journals including: Group Dynamics: Theory, Research & Practice, The Journal of Sport and Exercise Psychology, Small Group Research, The Journal of Behavioral Medicine, and Health Education and Behavior. Dr. Estabrooks' research is currently being supported by grants from the National Institutes of Health, USDA, and the Kansas Department of Health and Environment.

Dr. Richard D. Gordin is a professor at Utah State University. He is beginning his 21st year at the University. He is a professor in the department of health, physical education and recreation and is an adjunct professor in the department of psychology. He is also the graduate coordinator in the department. Dr. Gordin has published over 75 articles and book chapters and has made 300 professional presentations at regional, national, and international conferences. He has been a sport psychology consultant for numerous sports teams, including teams at his University, USA Gymnastics, USA Track and Field, US Fencing, and numerous professional golfers on the PGA Tour. He is the former chair of the certification committee of the Association for the Advancement of Applied Sport Psychology (AAASP). He is listed on the sport psychology registry of the United States Olympic Committee for the 2000-2004 quadrennium. He is also listed as a member of the USA Gymnastics Athlete Wellness program national referral network for 2001-2004. He has recently been appointed as one of the sport psychology consultants for USA Track and Field for the 2004 Olympic Games in Athens.

Peter Haberl, EdD, is employed as a sport psychology consultant in the sport science and coaching division of the USOC. In this position, he works with various resident teams and athletes at the Colorado Springs and Lake Placid Olympic Training Centers, providing individual and team consultations and counseling sessions on a daily basis. Peter accompanied USA Triathlon to the 2000 Summer Olympic Games in Australia. Now, the majority of his consulting work is focused on the mental preparation of the US Women's National and Olympic Ice Hockey Team for the 2002 Olympic Winter Games in Salt Lake City. Peter has been working as the sport psychology consultant for this team since 1996, attending the 1997, 1999, 2000, and 2001 World Championships. He frequently presents at coaching conventions and sport science conferences. Before entering his present position, Peter was a lecturer in sport psychology at Boston University where he completed his doctoral degree in counseling psychology with a specialization in sport psychology.

Tom Hanson, PhD has directed performance enhancement programs for the New York Yankees and the Texas Rangers. He has also consulted with the Anaheim Angels and Minnesota Twins and is co-author of Heads-Up Baseball: Playing the Game One Pitch at a Time. Hanson was head baseball coach and professor at Skidmore College (NY), where he worked with teams and athletes from a wide variety of sports. He was the hitting coach while earning his doctorate at the University of Virginia, and was a graduate assistant coach at the University of Illinois. For his research on the mental aspects of hitting, he interviewed Hank Aaron, Rod Carew, Tony Oliva, Pete Rose, Stan Musial, Billy Williams, Carl Yastrzemski, and Kirby Puckett. Hanson also has extensive experience coaching and training individuals and teams in the business world, specializing in CEOs and early stage companies. He resides in Tampa, Florida where he is CEO of Heads-Up Performance, Inc.

Barry Kirker is an Australasian psychologist, registered in Australia and New Zealand. He completed his applied Masters degree in sport and exercise psychology at the University of Southern Queensland, Australia in 1996, before consulting with teams and individuals from various sports and non-sporting organizations in Sydney, Australia. Barry completed his postgraduate thesis on aggression in team sport and has maintained a focus in this area, advising a number of professional rugby and soccer teams on how to manage player aggression. He has published journal articles and authored the chapter on sport psychology in the Oxford Handbook of Sports Medicine. He is currently a clinician in Auckland, New Zealand and is an active member of the New Zealand Sport Psychology Association and an accredited sport science provider to New Zealand's state-funded elite athletes.

Aidan Moran is professor of psychology, head of the department of psychology and director of the psychology research laboratory in University College, Dublin, Ireland. He is a Fulbright Scholar in cognitive psychology and has published extensively in peer-reviewed journals on such topics as attentional processes and mental imagery in athletes. Among his books are The Psychology of Concentration in Sport Performers: A Cognitive Analysis (1996, Psychology Press) and Managing Your Own Learning at University: A Practical Guide (1997, University College Dublin Press). He is a former official psychologist to the Irish Olympic Squad and is currently a consultant to many of Ireland's leading athletes and teams.

Tom Patrick is an instructor at the University of Winnipeg where he lectures on sport and exercise psychology, the organization and administration of sport and recreation, and current issues in the areas of physical activity and sport. He is the co-author of the book Human Potential: Perspective, Passion and Preparation, and has published a number of articles on various issues related to sport psychology and psychological skills training. Tom is also a certified consultant with the Canadian Mental Training Registry and has worked as a sport psychology consultant with numerous top international athletes and teams in both the United States and Canada. He is currently working with the Canadian National Women's Volleyball Team, the Canadian Racquetball Team, the National Swim Centre in Manitoba, the Manitoba National Triathlon Centre, and as an instructor with the National Coaching Institute in Manitoba. He is completing his doctoral studies at the University of Southern Queensland in Australia.

Ken Ravizza, PhD is a professor in the division of kinesiology and health promotion at Cal State University at Fullerton. He teaches courses in the areas of applied sport psychology, sport philosophy, and stress management. Ken served as the sport psychology consultant for the Anaheim Angels for fifteen years, and this year he made the move to the Los Angeles Dodgers. He works extensively with the Cal State Fullerton and Long Beach State baseball teams, and he has provided programs for the UCLA, LSU, Arkansas, USC, Texas, U Conn, and Harvard baseball teams. He has been a sport psychology consultant for the U.S. Olympic baseball, softball, field hockey, and water polo teams along with numerous individual Olympic athletes. In football he has worked with the University of Nebraska and the New York Jets. Ravizza has conducted over 100 sport psychology workshops nationally and internationally. His research includes examining the nature of peak performance in sport, and he is co-author of Heads-Up Baseball: Playing the Game One Pitch at a Time. He also sits on the editorial boards of the Sport Psychologist and Quest.

Robert "Bob" Singer has been on the faculty at different universities since receiving his PhD from Ohio State University, most notably Florida State University for 17 years and then the University of Florida for the last 14 years. He is chair of the department of exercise and sport sciences and has taught graduate classes and advised many doctoral students in topics related to motor learning and sport psychology. His research generally deals with cognitive processes and learner/performance strategies involved in skill acquisition and high levels of skill, and he has published over 100 research articles, over 200 scientific and professional articles, and 22 chapters in books. His last book publication, for which he is the lead co-editor, is the Handbook of Sport Psychology (2001, Wiley). It was his seventeenth book. Bob has served as head of the sport psychology division of the first Sports Medicine Committee of the United Stated Olympic Committee. Furthermore, Bob continues to consult with a number of athletes representing different sports. He has been elected president of the division of exercise and sport psychology of the American Psychological Association as well as president of the American Academy of Kinesiology and Physical Education. As president of the International Society of Sport Psychology (ISSP) for eight years, he was and still is actively involved in international developments and the advancement of sport psychology. He has made over 350 presentations in over 40 countries. Among many treasured recognitions, he received the Distinguished Contributions to the Science of Exercise of Sport and Exercise Psychology award in 1999 (the first of its kind), given by the division of exercise and sport psychology of the American Psychological Association, and the Distinguished International Sport Psychology award from the ISSP in 1997.

Gershon Tenenbaum is a professor at Florida State University. He is a former head of the centre of research and sport medicine sciences at the Wingate Institute in Israel (1982-1994) and the coordinator of the graduate program in sport and exercise psychology at the University of Southern Queensland in Australia (1994-1999). Gershon was the president of the International Society of Sport Psychology (ISSP) (1997-2001), and he is the editor of the International Journal of Sport Psychology. Gershon's areas of interest are in psychometrics, expertise (decision-making), and exertion tolerance. He has an extensive list of publications in journals and books and is a board member and reviewer for twelve scientific journals. He is a member of the Australia Psychological Society, College of Sport Psychology, New York Academy of Science, the American Society for the Advancement of Applied Science, North American Society of Sport and Physical Activity, the International Statistical Institute, and others. He received the ISSP Honor Award (1997), the USQ Researcher of the year (1997/1998), and the 1987 meritorious Contribution to Educational Research.

Ralph Vernacchia is a professor in the department of physical education, health and recreation at Western Washington University (Bellingham, WA, USA), where he directs the undergraduate and graduate programs in sport psychology and serves as the director of the Center for Performance Excellence. He is an AAASP fellow and certified consultant and a past chair of AAHPERD's Sport Psychology Academy. He is currently co-chair of USA Track and Field's sport psychology sub-committee, and has traveled internationally as a sport psychology consultant with several USA track and field teams, including the USA 2000 Olympic track and field team. He was a track and field coach for 22 years and has been inducted into the Western Washington University Athletic Hall of Fame in recognition of his coaching accomplishments.

Dr. Leonard D. Zaichkowsky has a BPE from the University of Alberta, an MED from the University of Oklahoma, and a PhD from the University of Toledo. Dr. Zaichkowsky's teaching and research specialty is the psychology of human development and performance. His current research interests include exercise and well-being, career transition of elite performers, development of expertise, and the psychophysiology of peak performance. Dr. Zaichkowsky has published over 50 articles on sport psychology and has co-authored or edited six books on motor development and sport psychology. He is a member of numerous state, national, and international organizations, including the Association for Applied Psychophysiology and Biofeedback, the American Psychological Association (APA), the International Society of Sport Psychology (ISSP), and the Association for the Advancement of Applied Sport Psychology (AAASP) (former president). Dr. Zaichkowsky is on the Registry of Sport Psychologists for the U.S. Olympic Committee and is the consulting sport psychologist for the Boston Celtics of the National Basketball Association.

INDEX

A

B

C